Early optimism surrounding the concept of community-based approaches to mental health care has frequently proved ill-founded. All too often community mental health care has merely resulted in rehousing people with long-term mental disorders in an alien community, where they remain as segregated from the real life of the community as if they were in large institutions.

This challenging book, based on the experience of the pioneering Buckingham project, a comprehensive mental health service focusing on primary care, describes a new approach to the provision of mental health service to a community. Taking as their theoretical basis the vulnerability–stress model of mental illness, the authors place their findings and recommendations in the wider context of mental health care provision, and draw widely on international research in this field. They insist on a rigorous approach to the provision and evaluation of care, and use telling case studies to reveal the benefits as well as some of the difficulties that may be experienced.

The practical, problem-solving and cost-effective approach described in this book will be of the greatest interest to health care professionals in whatever treatment-setting they may be working.

Integrated Mental Health Care

STUDIES IN SOCIAL AND COMMUNITY PSYCHIATRY

Volumes in this series examine the social dimensions of mental illness as they affect diagnosis and management, and address a range of fundamental issues in the development of community-based mental health services.

Series editor
PETER J. TYRER
Professor of Community Psychiatry, St Mary's Hospital Medical School, London

Integrated Mental Health Care

IAN R. H. FALLOON

Professor of Psychiatry
Chairman of Department of Psychiatry & Behavioural Science
University of Auckland, New Zealand

GRÁINNE FADDEN

Principal Clinical Psychologist
Buckingham Mental Health Service
Buckinghamshire, UK

and

Clinical Tutor
Oxford Regional Training Course in Clinical Psychology
Oxford, UK

Foreword by MICHAEL SHEPHERD

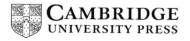
CAMBRIDGE
UNIVERSITY PRESS

Published by the Press Syndicate of the University of Cambridge
The Pitt Building, Trumpington Street, Cambridge CB2 1RP
40 West 20th Street, New York, NY 10011-4211, USA
10 Stamford Road, Oakleigh, Melbourne 3166, Australia

First published 1993

Printed in Great Britain
at the University Press, Cambridge

A catalogue record for this book is available from the British Library

Library of Congress cataloguing in publication data

Falloon, Ian R. H.
Integrated mental health care / Ian R. H. Falloon, Gráinne
Fadden.
     p.   cm.
Includes bibliographical references and index.
ISBN 0 521 39427 9 hardback
1. Buckingham Project.   2. Community psychiatry – England
– Case studies.   3. Community mental health services –
England – Administration – Case studies.   4. Community
mental health services – England – Evaluation – Case
studies.   I. Fadden, Gráinne.   II. Title.
   [DNLM: 1. Community Mental Health Services –
organization & administration – Great Britain.
WM 30 F196i]
RC455.F27   1992
362.2′0425′0942–dc20
DNLM/DLC
for Library of Congress   92–49810 CIP

ISBN 0 521 39427 9 hardback

PN

Contents

Foreword

During the past 30 years a new word, 'deinstitutionalisation', has come to signal a transition from the institutional to the extra-mural care of the mentally ill in Europe and North America. At the same time the complementary notion of 'community care' has become correspondingly fashionable despite the patently inadequate facilities available in most countries. In the 1980s the problems presented by the impending closure of British mental hospitals prompted an enquiry by a House of Commons Social Services Committee which commented pointedly on the 'virtually meaningless' nature of community care as a concept which had become little more than a slogan.[1] It is now apparent that, all too often, on leaving the protected environment of the asylum the psychiatric patient enters an environment in which care may be provided in some measure by community treatment as an extended form of hospital care but is given principally by formal and informal caregivers, among whom the medically qualified professional plays only one part. Who should this be?

The answer of the parliamentary committee was unequivocal: 'Community care depends to a large extent on the continuing capacity of GPs to provide primary medical care to mentally disabled people'. This view was first advanced in Britain on the basis of research conducted nearly 30 years ago.[2] It reflects the findings of many studies carried out since then and supports the conclusion of a World Health Organisation report, that 'the primary care team is the cornerstone of community psychiatry'.[3] In acknowledging the fact that the bulk of mental illness in any community never comes to the attention of a psychiatric specialist, however, it also brings a radically different perspective to community psychiatry, one which employs a socio-medical approach within a public health framework. Teamwork becomes indispensable, and the general practitioner's activities extend to close collaboration with non-medical colleagues, especially social workers, nurses and psychologists. And by the same token the role of the psychiatrist is diminished. In Australia, despite a different system of medical care, a Quality Assurance Project has reached similar conclusions: 'It is now evident that the majority of persons who meet criteria for a mental disorder and who seek treatment will be treated by a health professional other than a psychiatrist'.[4]

To outline the situation defined by research findings is one thing. To translate them into action is another. The basic problem, as a professor of social policy has pointed out, is that 'we do not yet have a clear organisation model for the community mental health services as a whole, or the political will to produce one'.[5] The task calls for energy, imagination and resourcefulness, and in attempting to create a model service in an English rural area, Dr. Falloon and his colleagues have broken new ground. In this book the authors present a detailed account of the background, origins and development of the Buckingham Project and some of the early findings. Their work merits the close attention of everyone with an interest in the future prospects of care for the mentally ill.

Michael Shepherd, CBE, DM, FRCP, FRCPsych(Hon) DPM
Emeritus Professor of Epidemiological Psychiatry

[1] House of Commons Social Services Committee (1965): *Community care.* H.M.S.O., London (Second Report).
[2] Shepherd M., Cooper B., Brown A.C. & Kalton G.W. (1966) *Psychiatric illness in general practice.* Oxford University Press, London.
[3] World Health Organisation Working Groups (1973) *Psychiatry and Primary Medical Care.* W.H.O., Copenhagen.
[4] Andrews G. (1991) The changing nature of psychiatry. *Australian and New Zealand Journal of Psychiatry,* **25**, 453–459.
[5] Jones K. (1992) Review of 'community psychiatry: the principles'. *British Journal of Psychiatry,* **160**, 138–139.

Preface

This book outlines a new concept in mental health care that was conceived nearly thirty years ago by Professor Michael Shepherd, when he noted that most people who experienced episodes of mental disorders received little care from the specialist hospital-based mental health services, and were managed, for the most part successfully, within the primary care sector. Since that time many attempts have been made to integrate aspects of specialist mental health services with those of primary care. However, these efforts tended to focus on specific specialties, such as psychiatric consultation, psychological treatment, social casework or community psychiatric nursing. This book describes the development of a service that fully integrates a comprehensive mental health team within a primary care setting. All the specialist services associated with hospital-based care are provided within the primary care framework.

The Buckingham project began in March 1984 when the Oxford Regional Health Authority agreed to appoint a Consultant Physician in Mental Health in the Northern area of the Aylesbury Vale. He was given the remit to develop a model mental health service to a semi-rural area that covered approximately 200 square miles between the cities of Aylesbury and Oxford to the South, Milton Keynes on the West, Banbury on the East and Northampton to the North. This area is mainly farmland, with small towns and villages scattered throughout. The close proximity to the M1 and M40 motorways and to railway services to London's Euston and Paddington stations makes it an increasingly attractive area for commuters. The current population of 35,000 is expected to almost double by the turn of the century, making it one of the most rapidly growing areas in Europe. More than half the population live in the towns of Buckingham and Winslow. Buckingham is an historic town, until the end of last century the County Town of Buckinghamshire. It has tended to maintain its traditions of excellent services, with a good range of shopping facilities, schools and health care resources, including a 15-bedded community hospital, that provides a full range of outpatient clinics and basic casualty services.

The service was funded from savings made from the Aylesbury Vale District Health Authority and Buckinghamshire Social Services development funds. From small beginnings, when staffing consisted of 14 family practitioners, 11 community nurses (4 district nurses, 4 health visitors, 2 midwives and 1 practice nurse) the psychiatrist and a half-time psychiatric nurse, the service expanded to a staff of 18 family practitioners, 12 community nurses, 12 mental health nurses, 1 clinical psychologist, 1 occupational therapist, 1 social worker, 2 psychiatrists and three administrative staff. The specialist mental health personnel represented the total staff allocation for a 15-bedded hospital unit with 15 day hospital places that had been planned for the Buckingham area. This new unit opened in 1990, by which time the community-based service had become fully operational and no longer needed extensive hospital-based provisions. As a result the community was able to use the purpose-built unit primarily for general medical care, which included infrequent use for people with mental disorders requiring special care that could not be provided at home.

The support of a forward thinking senior management contributed to this enterprise. Major personal commitments of Dame Rosemary Rue, Drs Ian Yule, Julian Pedley, David Watt, Christopher Brown, Ms Rosemary Pritchard and Mrs Janice Miles facilitated the early and continued development of the project. Valuable consultation was provided on the clinical developments by Drs John Hoult, Loren Mosher, Richard Lamb, Leonard Stein and Douglas Bennett. An evaluation team was developed at an early stage, supported by funds from the Mental Health Foundation, the Oxford Regional Research Fund, and the Department of Health. Support from Professors Michael Shepherd, Michael Gelder, Robert Liberman, and Drs John Reed and Rachel Jenkins was generously provided to assist in developing the service evaluation methods employed. In more recent times a training and dissemination project has been developed with the support of funds from Research and Development in Psychiatry, under the leadership of Professor Tom Craig.

However, the major contributors to the success of this project were the staff of the service itself, who were among the most committed, enthusiastic and talented people one could wish to meet. Their willingness to work in a highly flexible manner, to eagerly learn new ways to manage mental disorders, to help one another, was an inspiration to all who came in contact with them. All those wonderful people are acknowledged on pages xvi–xvii. However, one or two warrant special mentions: Terry Pembleton, a nurse with outstanding commitment to patients and staff alike; Bridget Lake, an occupational therapist, who always seemed to be able to find time to assist anyone in need; Kay Mehrtens, a social worker, who facilitated excellent liaison between the service and a wide range of social resources in the community; Hazel King, an administrative secretary, with exceptional interpersonal skills; and Victor Graham-Hole and Lynne Norris, two cognitive-behavioural nurse therapists who insisted on maintaining a service of the highest quality at all times. These people were the foundation upon which the integrated approach to mental health care was built. The combined efforts of all the staff allowed an exceptional teamwork approach to develop that impressed observers from all parts of the globe. However, such cohesive teamwork presented a problem for new staff and trainees, who found it difficult to readjust to the highly efficient, competent and confident approach that was prevalent. Once this problem was recognised special efforts were made to assist new members to integrate, through the preparation of detailed guidebooks and manuals and attendance at practical training courses.

This book is the culmination of these efforts to define the key elements of integrated mental health care in a straightforward and practical sense. The attempt to match theory with practice and to measure the outcome is documented. It is hoped that this will give clinicians and academics a clear picture of the approach so that they may be able to develop services along similar principles, and achieve similar benefits. To date the integrated care approach has been fully deployed in only one service, but over 50 services have utilised several of the main components, and many are endeavouring to incorporate all the elements into their community-based developments. The precise structure of the services is likely to differ according to local needs and resources. However, it is crucial that all modern mental health services are based upon empirical evidence for the effectiveness and efficiency of specific clinical management strategies and that all mental health professionals are trained as scientist-practitioners. Only then will our field receive appropriate recognition for the outstanding contribution it makes to enhancing the quality of life of our communities. This scientific approach should not be equated with cold, calculated manipulation of peoples thoughts and emotions, but with the warm humanity of committed practitioners who provide accessible, acceptable and adaptable approaches to care to all who will benefit. This book describes one such attempt to provide such a service.

I.R.H. Falloon
G. Fadden

Buckingham project staff

Dr Peter Atherton
Patrick Beale
Caroline Birch
Dr Christopher Brown
Dr Judith Burgess
David Callinan
Dr Julian Candy
Dr Iain Clark
Dr Peter Cohen
Audrey Cornwall
Harry Darku
June Dent
Dr Elizabeth Dickson
Dr Roger Dickson
Patrick Dignam
Gráinne Fadden
Dr Ian Falloon
Edward Fitzgerald
Dr Valerie Foster-Smith
Victor Graham-Hole
Natalie Hall
Ian Hall-Scott
Dr Roger Harrington
Ian Heath
Marie Kelly
Hazel King
Dr Haroutyan Krekorian
Bridget Lake
Dr Marc Laporta
Roger Lim-Hon
Dr Stephen Logsdail
Dr Richard Marsh

Dr Rebecca Mather
Dr Stuart Mathews
Sheila McLees
Jacob Mensa
Kay Mehrtens
Dr Claire Monaghan
Martina Mueller
John Mullis
Lesley Mulroy
Leona Murray
Lynne Norris
Lesley Park
Terry Pembleton
Dr Collin Place
Leah Ray
Lady Marjorie Reid (deceased)
Dr Diana Riley
Dr Elaine Robb
Jennifer Roberts
Dr William Shanahan
Anita Silver
Dr Michael Spencer
Dr Phillip Stowell
Brenda Stroud
Dr Richard Thomas
Julie Uglow
Dr David Watt
Professor Greg Wilkinson
Dr Ian Wood
Janice Wright
Dr Robert Woodroffe

and all the Community Nursing and Administrative staff of Buckingham, Steeple Claydon and Winslow Districts and Buckingham Hospital

1

Introduction: who needs community-based care?

In recent years the development of community-based approaches to mental health services has become encumbered by ideological concerns that have obscured the simple reality of service provision. The term 'community' has been used as a battle cry for a revolution against the tyranny attributed to the medical model, while the emphasis on *mental health* has led to a focus on the provision of scarce health care resources to enhance the general well-being of all persons living in conditions of social deprivation or personal distress, and the subsequent provision of little more than tea-and-chat for those ravaged by major mental disorders. The high expectations that a move away from the Victorian mental asylums to new surroundings in the middle of urban settings would lead to rapid recovery of functioning and a healthy and productive lifestyle have seldom been sustained. Such ill-informed optimism has often led to the recreation of the same deprivation found in the institutions, particularly when the enthusiasm of the reformers has been tempered by the realisation that serious mental disorders are not cured merely by human warmth and understanding (Lamb & Goertzel, 1970). All too often community mental health has merely resulted in rehousing people with long-term mental disorders in an alien community, where they remain as segregated from the real life of the community as much as they were in the large institutions – men and women of the shadows, easy prey for the streetwise, and frequent victims of inadequate health, social and legal systems.

There are exceptions to this model of relocating hospital-based practices to dispersed urban sites. Unfortunately, relatively few of these models have become generally accepted. All require a considerable investment in the development of well-trained, professional staff, who have the skills to conduct comprehensive state-of-the-art clinical management of clearly defined mental disorders in all settings within the community. Professional staff need to be committed to working with people with long-standing and multiple difficulties, where progress is often extremely slow and lacks the immediate rewards associated with acute care and crisis intervention with people suffering from stressful life events. Furthermore, recent advances in the delivery of community-based mental health services have tended to be based upon a careful analysis of the lifestyle of the individual within his or her social network. This allows adaptations to be made that minimise the handicaps associated with persisting disability in those chronically impaired or vulnerable to recurrences. Such an ecological analysis of the human habitat has been largely ignored by hospital-based approaches to mental health services, where concern has focussed merely on providing an acceptable institutional environment for intensive treatment. This book will attempt to describe an approach to the provision of comprehensive mental health services to a community, which integrates the benefits of biological psychiatry with recent developments in psychological and social interventions that aim to minimise all forms of morbidity associated with mental disorders.

An evaluative model for the development and evaluation of a mental health service to a community

The successful provision of a service to a community is one that meets all the relevant needs for that community with maximal efficacy and at minimal costs, both economic and emotional. Raeburn and Seymour (1977) proposed an excellent model of a systematic approach to the planning, implementation and evaluation of a service that we have adapted as a guide to this development (Figure 1.1). The steps provide a guide not merely to the development and maintenance of the service, but also provide a parallel guide for the development of therapeutic management strategies for individual cases.

The first step in service development entails an accurate *assessment of the current needs of a defined population* for the relevant service. The

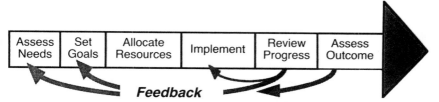

Figure 1.1. A co-ordinated strategy for planning a service based upon meeting the needs of the community served. (From Raeburn & Seymour, 1977.)

more specifically the needs can be defined in terms of specific types of impairments, disabilities and handicaps associated with mental disorders, as well as the incidence, prevalence and severity of this morbidity, the more accurately appropriate resources can be estimated with which to resolve these problems.

An important intermediate step involves *setting goals for the service* so that resources are allocated efficiently to achieve clearly defined priorities which are closely related to identified needs. Goals need to be clearly defined, realistic and readily assessed. Disorders for which no current therapeutic strategies are available may necessitate quite different goals to preventable or curable conditions. However, it is crucial that every significant area of need is targeted, not merely those with a special appeal to the service providers, or those that are currently topical as a result of political or economic consequences; e.g. services for child abuse, homelessness, unemployment, or the psychological effects of war and disasters.

The allocation of resources is conducted in a manner that enables achievement of the specific goals of the service in the most efficient manner. Where resources are clearly insufficient to provide effective interventions to achieve all the goals, priorities may need to be set and more limited goals targeted in the early stages. We would propose that the criteria upon which such decisions are founded are based on levels of severity of the impairment, disability and handicaps of individuals and the resultant distress they experience. Efficient utilisation of resources may enable additional goals, of lower priority, to be tackled later. However, where high priority goals remain despite efficient deployment of the resources currently

allocated, planning must ensure that the necessary additional resources are secured at the earliest possible time. A careful assessment of the resources that are available within a community may
reveal substantial hidden assets that have not been fully utilised by
traditional hospital-based services, but may be readily accessible to
a community-based service. A survey of community resources is a
vital component of service development.

The *implementation* step entails application of the technology that is
most cost-effective in the achievement of the service goals. In mental
health services this usually involves training staff in those therapeutic skills which have been proven to be effective in treating the
disorders whose alleviation they have defined as the specific service
goals. A secondary consideration would appear to be the setting in
which these skills are applied, particularly issues of bricks-and-
mortar. In many cases the location of treatment is crucial to the
effective and efficient application of therapeutic skills. All too often
planning produces the situation where the persons with the greatest
technical expertise are located in places where they can apply that
expertise in the least effective manner, and persons with less technical skill are located in settings where technical expertise is most
beneficial. For example, relatively unskilled nursing staff are frequently burdened with the care of the most disabled, while highly
skilled psychologists and psychiatrists spend disproportionate
amounts of time working with persons who are much less disabled.
This has been a major problem in the devolution of hospital-based
services and the development of community-based methods. Such
activity is often labelled as prevention, but there is little evidence
that primary prevention of major mental disorders is effective
(Lamb & Zusman, 1981), whereas early detection and intervention
of major disorders may prevent long-term disability and handicap in
persons who develop these conditions. It makes sense to target
valuable and usually scarce resources to those cases where mental
health specialists can provide the expert skills that are lacking within
existing community resources.

Regular and continuous *evaluation of the manner in which therapeutic
skills are implemented* is a crucial aspect of a service. A method of
assessing the progress of every case, as well as specific groups of
impairments, disabilities or handicaps is essential. Such methods
should reflect change accurately, be readily applied in the clinical

setting, and processed in an efficient manner so that therapists and managers alike can make use of the feedback to adjust strategies on a day-to-day basis.

Major *service reviews* should be conducted on a less frequent basis, usually annually. These reviews should indicate whether the goals have been achieved and the community needs met by the service. They may also indicate whether the process of resource allocation and implementation has been efficient. Such feedback enables the constructive revision of goals to enhance the efficiency of the service in meeting all the changing needs of the community it serves.

Defining the needs of a community

Perhaps the most important step in establishing a service to a community is the ability to pinpoint the needs of that community for that particular service. Ideally the assessment of the needs of a service should be based upon a series of community surveys of the incidence and prevalence of all forms of mental disorder and their related disabilities and handicaps. Such surveys are very expensive and are seldom feasible in clinical practice. Moreover, from the moment a staff member is appointed to provide a clinical service in a community setting it is likely that the service is deemed open for business and that person is expected to meet all the needs of the community forthwith. This is in stark contrast to new hospital services, where the delays associated with building and equipping the hospital enable staff to be hired to plan the service, receive training and fully prepare themselves for the initial intake of patients when the hospital unit opens.

It is unfortunate that it is seldom possible to define local needs for mental health services in an ideal fashion through epidemiological surveys. However, it is not the only method of gaining information about community needs and several alternative methods may be considered. These include: reviewing the literature on the incidence and prevalence of mental disorders in epidemiological surveys conducted in demographically similar areas; examining the cases currently known to the hospital-based services; examining the cases currently known to the primary care services, both medical and social. The last may include a survey of all persons receiving psychotropic drugs.

Fortunately, a number of excellent community surveys of the prevalence of mental disorders have been conducted in recent years. These surveys provide a good guide to the likely needs of a community for the clinical management of established mental disorders. The recent development of standardised diagnostic schedules and sophisticated epidemiological methods (Regier et al, 1985) has enabled us to generalise from these studies to a much greater extent than before. The two most comprehensive surveys, one in five urban settings in the United States (Regier et al, 1984), the other in rural Bavaria (Dilling & Weyerer, 1984), suggest that, at least in industrialised countries, the prevalence of the major mental disorders is strikingly similar. Although there is evidence that in non-industrialised cultures the pattern of recovery from mental disorders differs substantially from that of the industrialised world (Sartorius et al, 1977), it seems reasonable to plan community services on the basis of this epidemiological data. It may be important to note that there is no evidence that the prevalence of mental disorders is lower in rural areas, although severely handicapped persons, particularly those complicated with the additional problems of substance abuse and personality disorders, tend to aggregate in those inner city areas where cheap housing and medical and social agencies can be accessed without lengthy and expensive travel (Faris & Dunham, 1939; Hafner & Reimann, 1970).

Epidemiological surveys of mental health problems in Britain have been devoted mainly to examining the patterns of consultation with the well-developed primary care services (Goldberg & Huxley, 1980; Shepherd et al, 1966). The data derived from these studies do not include the substantial proportion of the mentally disordered who do not attend their family practitioners. It is sometimes assumed that the population that are missed in such surveys includes only persons with minor conditions, but it is likely that a substantial proportion of persons with serious mental disorders do not seek help from medical services (Goldberg & Huxley, 1980). One paradox concerning persons with serious mental disorders is that, unlike most sufferers of physical disorders, they tend to avoid contact with medical services. An even larger proportion of cases who attend their general practitioners are not recognised as suffering from mental disorders. These are frequently people who present with physical complaints of anxiety or depressive disorders and pose

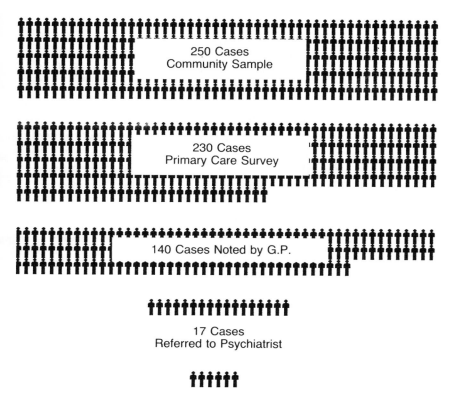

Figure 1.2. One-year prevalence of mental disorders per 1,000 population when observed from a variety of sampling methods. (From Goldberg & Huxley, 1980.)

considerable detection problems for sophisticated assessors (Goldberg & Bridges, 1987). Finally, relatively few of those who are recognised as suffering from mental disorders by their family doctors are sent for specialist consultations, and even fewer are admitted to inpatient units. This series of 'filters' through which patients must pass to receive intensive mental health care from hospital-based services is summarised in Figure 1.2.

This schematic representation of the prevalence of mental disorders in the community, illustrated in Figure 1.2, has many striking features. One in four of the adult population will suffer a definable mental disorder during the course of a year, i.e. 20,000 per 100,000; of whom 3000–5000 are deemed severe cases requiring specialist services, and 300–500 will benefit from 24-hour intensive treatment at any time. On this basis the provision of hospital beds and outpatient services would have to be increased at least 10-fold to meet the community's needs, even in areas where such services currently are considered sufficient. Hidden morbidity that is not receiving specialist services presents a major problem that must be considered in the development of community-based services.

It is evident that there is a major discrepancy in this estimate of service need. The explanations for this discrepancy are not clear. Two possible explanations may be considered. First, current models of hospital-based services are developed primarily to manage persons suffering from the functional psychoses (mainly schizophrenia and major affective disorders). These conditions are often episodic and have a relatively low prevalence in the community. Severe anxiety disorders, dysthymic states, and stress response syndromes, tend to have high levels of disability and handicap, often persist over long periods, but are not thought to benefit from hospital care. Indeed, the main criteria for admission to a mental hospital is not merely the severity of morbidity, but more often the levels of distress the patient engenders in those with whom he or she has contact with in the community. Thus, admission is often sought after a social crisis by persons other than the patient (Wing, 1968). The mental hospital retains much of its asylum role, albeit not solely for the patient.

The second hypothesis is that for many people who are seriously impaired, 24-hour intensive treatment is provided already in settings other than hospitals, mainly through informal care in their own homes. Families and friends combined with the professional support of the primary care teams – family doctors, community nurses and social workers – provide effective intensive treatment which often matches that provided in the best hospital units. Evidence to support this hypothesis is discussed in greater detail in Chapter 2.

The identification of all those who would benefit from mental health management in a community must account not merely for those cases that are already known to the hospital-based and primary care services, but also for those cases who have not yet been recognised by the professional services or have been misclassified by those services. This presents a major dilemma for service planning.

A survey of all cases known to the services, including all discharges from those services in the previous five years, might uncover cases that have already been detected, but this leaves considerable hidden morbidity. Improved screening by family practitioners, community nurses and social service workers would address some aspects of this problem, but a significant minority of severely disabled persons may remain undetected in the community. A survey of all patients receiving psychoactive drugs may lead to detection of other hidden cases. Attempts at increasing community awareness and increasing consumer support for the mental health service may facilitate uptake of services by those currently reluctant to seek assistance from services widely publicised for their failings rather than their successes. Although there is no research to guide planning, securing the support of local organisations and particularly the local media, may be expected to assist in publicising the existence of new consumer-oriented services.

Reliable and valid assessment of mental disorders is crucial in the definition of the population that a mental health service is contracted to serve. Research-based studies have contributed to the development of sophisticated diagnostic classification of mental disorders, so that high levels of agreement between clinicians can be obtained where standardised diagnostic interviews and classification systems are used (Sartorius et al, 1977). Less well developed, but of equal importance, are methods to assess the levels of impairment, disability and handicap associated with mental disorders. Diagnostic classification provides minimal guidance to the morbidity and quality of life experienced by persons suffering from mental disorders, or the secondary morbidity associated with their care. A comprehensive assessment of the needs of a community for mental health services should include measures of impairment, disability and handicap of sufferers and informal carers (Table 1.1.).

Impairment refers to the pathophysiological interference with bodily functions that characterises various mental disorders and produces the symptoms of each disorder. In the absence of clear evidence of underlying pathology for most mental disorders, the impairments of mental disorders are characterised mainly by their phenomenological features. Thought interference, perceptual distortion, motor abnormality and impaired information processing are all found in most major disorders. The level of such disturbance provides a measure of the severity of impairment of the disorder.

Table 1.1. *Impairment, disability and handicap*

Impairments	Disabilities	Handicaps
Thought interference	Cognitive:	Lack of friends
Perceptual distortion	inefficient problem solving,	Unemployment
Motor abnormality	slowed learning	Limited leisure
Reduced attention span	Affective:	activity
Reduced drive	inappropriate fear, feelings	Poor housing and
Impaired information	of inadequency	self-care
processing	Behavioural:	Carers burdened
	low rate of constructive	
	actions	

Such measures are not well developed and tend to be derived from diagnostic interview schedules by summing the total number of symptoms reported (Wing et al, 1974). A few scales of global severity of mental disorders have been developed, but their standardisation is limited (Guy, 1976). As research into the pathology of mental disorders progresses, it is anticipated that physiological abnormalities will provide clearer indices of the levels of severity of mental disorders to support our clinical observations.

Disability refers to the disturbances in functioning that are associated with the impairments of mental disorders. Slowed learning, inefficient problem solving, inappropriate affective responses and reductions in constructive activities are among the disabilities commonly associated with mental disorders. It is clear that such disturbances can be manifestations of many other conditions and are not specific to mental disorders. Further, they represent the psychological impact of impairment upon a person's functioning and can be measured by psychological assessments of cognition, affect and behaviour. Psychological coping mechanisms may help an individual compensate for these disabilities, so that some people with limited personal coping resources will be incapacitated by relatively mild levels of impairment, whereas others, with good coping abilities will be able to compensate for severe impairments. For example, one person who experienced occasional disruptions from auditory hallucinations remained extremely anxious, with profound feelings of inadequacy, leading to gross social withdrawal, while a second person continued to pursue a career as a writer and to engage in a wide range of social activities, despite frequent interruption of his thought processes by similar hallucinations.

Handicap refers to the disturbance in social functioning that is associated with disability. Difficulties with work, companionship, leisure, recreation, and self-care are some of the handicaps associated with mental disorders. Once again, an individual with good premorbid psychosocial development will be less prone to develop major handicaps from his or her disorder, whereas people from deprived backgrounds will most readily succumb. The provision of social case management to assist individuals, as well as the communities in which they live, to adapt to their disabilities is likely to contribute to reductions in handicaps. However, the concept of handicap extends beyond the individual to those people in the community who are involved in caring for the disabled. The limitations placed upon the personal and social lives of carers should be considered carefully when conducting a comprehensive assessment of the community needs associated with mental disorders. Standardised measures of handicaps often confuse handicap and disability. For example, a person who is not employed may well be able to work in a low stress work environment, but is handicapped where such jobs are not available in the local workforce. Similarly, a person living in a rural community may have little opportunity to continue education or to engage in a range of recreational pursuits.

To conclude, a comprehensive review of the needs of a community for mental health services should extend beyond the detection of cases of mental disorder to include the assessment of impairment, disability and handicap associated with those persons and their informal carers.

Definition of the goals of mental health services

The goals of most mental health services are poorly defined. In the absence of clear goals, services are often defined by the nature of the cases referred to them. Such lack of specificity leads to inevitable failure, with referral agents tending to use the service less for specialist consultation, and more as a means to reduce their own anxiety and frustrations with the care of difficult cases, many of whom have needs outside the remit of the service. As mentioned

earlier, requests for patients to be admitted to mental hospitals tend
to relate as much to the social needs of the community caregivers as
to the need for intensive medical assessment and treatment (Wing,
1968; Parkes, 1978). Warner (1985) has demonstrated an association between admission rates to mental hospitals and periods of
economic recession when unemployment is high and housing in
short supply. Mental hospitals have long provided a respite from the
social stresses of the community and as a result have become an
important provider of 24-hour *social care and emergency housing* for the
community. The closure of a mental hospital tends to place more
burdens on the social services, particularly the housing resources,
than on the medical services, and the term *rehabilitation* is often
employed as a euphemism for *rehousing*. Therefore, it is not surprising
that such sleight of hand creates considerable tensions between
agencies and contributes to resistance to such changes.

For the purposes of legitimising hospital admission, medical
labels are readily applied to persons suffering from distressing social
problems. They are 'anxious', 'depressed', 'hopeless', 'confused',
'distraught', 'agitated' and 'suicidal'. Without the application of
clear definitions for mental disorders, or for the criteria for entry into
specialist mental health services, abuse is frequent. It may be easy to
criticise cases of blatant political abuse in totalitarian states, while
remaining blind to the more subtle misuse of mental hospitals in less
restrictive cultures. Our services should be *primarily* for the benefit of
the index patient, who is suffering from a clearly defined mental
disorder, and *secondarily* for the benefit of family members or professional community caregivers. In a survey of 18 patients admitted
to hospital units during the first year of the new Buckingham service,
only two were admitted expressly for specific medical treatment.
The remainder were admitted almost entirely for social reasons.

It is crucial that the goals of a mental health service are tailored to
the specific needs of all mentally disordered persons residing in that
community, as well as those identified as having a high risk of
developing major mental disorders. This must include efforts to
prevent mental disorders, particularly those serious disorders that
tend to become chronic, as well as to provide the best treatment
available to all persons who do succumb to mental disorders. Such
efforts would seek to achieve the ultimate goal of reducing the
prevalence of mental disorders in the community and the disabilities
and handicaps that result from these disorders.

Table 1.2. *Aims of an integrated mental health service*

To support existing competent primary care services
To supplement primary care with efficient specialised strategies
To reduce impairment, disability and handicaps associated with all mental
  disorders, including that incurred by informal and professional caregivers
To integrate all mental health care in a community
To facilitate accessibility and acceptability of mental health care to all members
  of the community
To ensure that every person in the community receives the optimal clinical
  management of their disorders

The goals of such a service are summarised in Table 1.2. This service aims to integrate primary and specialist mental health care so that all those people suffering as a result of mental disorders can receive optimal clinical management, not merely those who have been traditionally within the ambit of hospital care. Such goals may seem highly unrealistic for a service that is planned according to hospital-based models. However, as we shall see later in this chapter, feasibility improves when we view the problem from a community-based perspective.

Integrated biopsychosocial case management of all people who are suffering from established mental disorders is an essential goal. This ensures that at all times each person receives the clinical management needed to minimise the morbidity associated with his or her mental disorder until full recovery from all impairment, disability and handicaps has been sustained for a minimum of two years, and many remain in long-term management indefinitely. The concept of dropping out of the service is not accepted. The readiness of many mental health professionals to label people as 'non-compliant', 'refusers' or 'drop-outs' often reflects their unwillingness to put in the effort needed to engage effectively those people with complex difficulties, or those whose current reluctance is the result of their previous experiences of not receiving adequate help in the past. Non-compliance with clinical management plans becomes just another problem to be addressed. The service actively pursues interventions that seek to ensure that optimal treatment is provided continuously in a manner that proves acceptable to each person according to their individual needs. Intensive management continues throughout the different phases of the disorder. This includes the provision of 24-hour interventions during the acute phases, as well as day, evening and weekend treatment sessions during rehabilitation.

Many family members of disabled persons suffer from mental disorders themselves. They may be more vulnerable to specific mental disorders as a result of shared genetic and environmental factors, which are prone to be triggered by the added stress of caring for a person with a mental disorder, or any excessive stress to the household environment from manifestations of the disabled person's disorder. Thus, a high priority goal is to include every household member in the clinical management plan, with their specific mental health needs addressed on a long-term basis in a similar fashion to that of the disabled person. In other words, individuals are never managed in isolation, but within the framework of a care unit that involves at least one informal carer. In addition, the needs of professional caregivers should also be considered, so that their health can be maintained at optimal levels and their case management efforts sustained in a manner that maximises long-term implementation of care.

Not all persons suffering from psychosocial disturbance are considered within the primary ambit of mental health services. Many persons display disability and handicap identical to those associated with mental disorders. Examples include interpersonal difficulties, poor social skills, inefficient problem solving, antisocial behaviour patterns, lack of motivation or poor vocational achievement. However, if there is no evidence that these deficits are the sequelae of the specific impairment of a mental disorder, such persons are not considered legitimate primary targets for a mental health service that is contracted to attend to the needs of the large proportion of the community who are suffering from clearly defined mental disorders. However, many of the psychosocial interventions that are effective in the management of mental disorders are also indicated for these psychological and social problems. In such instances the goal of the mental health service is to ensure that the person receives the most effective treatment for his or her condition through the most appropriate community agency. Training and consultation for other professionals and voluntary agencies in psychosocial intervention skills is advocated, rather than taking over their roles in the community.

The final goal is to develop a method of providing continuous feedback on all aspects of the delivery of service. This enables the strengths and weaknesses to be readily identified and constructive changes to be instigated at the earliest possible time so that the service remains sensitive to the changing needs of the consumers. Simplistic feedback on the numbers of persons admitted or discharged, the case loads of therapists, or the utilisation of hospital places, are poor indicators of the quality of the case management that is provided. Efforts to develop straightforward measures that enable levels of clinical, social and economic benefits and needs to be constantly monitored have been one of the key goals of the service. Once again it is crucial that the service is designed in a manner that permits the knowledge of results to rapidly induce change in practice.

Allocation of resources

Health services are usually planned by allocating resources primarily on the basis of the hospital facilities needed for a given catchment population, rather than on the specific needs of the community that is served. As we have argued earlier in this chapter, only a small proportion of mental health services to communities are delivered by traditional hospital services. Thus, where services are planned from a hospital-based perspective, there is a serious danger that the allocation of resources will be skewed, with most of the resources being used to manage few of the community needs. An effective service to a community can only be achieved where resources are allocated according to need, and in view of the constant change of that need, such allocation must be highly flexible. Institutional resources, such as hospitals, outpatient clinics and day treatment centres are seldom able to provide this flexibility even when intervention programmes are targeted towards individual goals. At best they probably meet half the population's needs half the time.

Regardless of the manner in which resources are appropriated for a service, it is vital that they are adequate to meet the needs of the community to be served, although there is accumulating evidence that the incidence of mental disorders is quite similar in most parts of the world and in different social settings. However, the prevalence of major mental disorders and their associated levels of disability and handicap undoubtedly differ according to social circumstances. Despite this, in almost every instance staff allocation for publicly

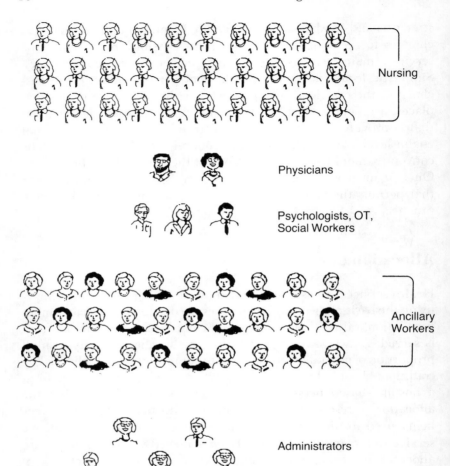

Figure 1.3. The hospital-based team that provides the basic resource allocated for British mental health service developments.

funded mental health services is based upon simple population data alone. The typical pattern of staff for a mental health service is depicted in Figure 1.3. This is based upon the assumption that the service will replicate a hospital-based team in some manner. Thus, staff posts consist of a large number of nurses, most of whom have few skills relevant to meeting the needs of the community, where family members and other informal carers happily perform many of the roles accorded to nurses in institutional settings. The remaining staff posts consist of a small number of other professions to provide consultation to the nurses. The large number of non-professional staff who provide institutional support for a hospital-based service including the 'hotel' services, including cooking, cleaning, gardening, electrical and maintenance work, are seldom considered in the development of a community-based service, although their expertise could provide substantial support if deployed in the community to support sufferers and carers in their homes. Thus, skilful planning is required to deploy a team of professional mental health workers and ancillary staff in a manner that maximises their ability to meet the mental health needs of the community in an optimal way.

While the major resource for mental health services is skilled professional staff, the provision of resources to accommodate staff in appropriate locations in the community and the need for specialised accommodation and resources to meet the needs of the sufferers and carers must be addressed. In planning a community-based service, it is crucial that such resources should be allocated according to the clearly defined needs of the consumers, not the expressed needs of the mental health professionals. The emphasis should be on the ready accessibility of a team of skilled professionals to all persons suffering from mental disorders in the community and their caregivers. This should be done in a manner that facilitates the provision of optimal clinical management and expedites rapid, sustained recovery from all impairment, disability and handicaps. Such planning begins and ends with people in their natural habitats. Any attempt to remove them to other locations, such as hospitals, clinics, day centers, etc. should be carefully considered in terms of the advantages and disadvantages of such removal to the consumers. The costs, both emotional and economic, of specialised institutional resources need to be weighed against the alternative approach of meeting the consumers' needs in a highly individualised manner that uses the highly specialised, group-oriented hospital resources as an essential back-up to the well-resourced community-based service. This is in contrast to the more traditional system of using the hospital as the major source of specialised clinical management, supported by a token community service providing follow-up care. To date few public health services have been willing to provide adequate resources to establish both up-to-date hospital-based and community-based services, so that careful choices must be made about the focus of the service. We argue throughout this book that a fully equipped community-based service, supported by a highly specialised hospital service is more effective in meeting community needs than an extensive hospital-based service that is supported by a highly specialised community service. In this model resources are initially provided to the community-based development, which when fully deployed may be expected to minimise the need for traditional hospital-based services, and define those needs in terms of highly specialised units to deal with very complex biopsychosocial problems, using highly sophisticated intensive management procedures that are currently available only in a few research-based units.

Epidemiological surveys that have examined the way that mental health services were already being provided in the absence of sophisticated specialist services have shown that most cases are receiving adequate clinical management already (Dilling & Weyerer, 1984; Goldberg & Huxley, 1980). It is evident that in most communities there is already a highly effective network of community-based services operating. This is made up first and foremost, by patients and their caregivers, mainly families, who endeavour to manage a wide range of mental disorders. These include some extremely severe chronic cases, who present considerable management difficulties when they present to hospital-based services, and have often opted out of such services. When asked why they chose to shoulder the burdens such care entailed, caregivers in Buckingham reported that the hospital was too far away, and had not helped them much in the past when their relatives had been admitted for treatment. Their family doctors tended to echo these sentiments and seemed willing to provide drugs and support for these persons without specialist consultation. These findings are similar to those found in research surveys (Shepherd et al, 1966; Dilling & Weyerer, 1984).

In addition to the informal and primary care services, many communities have been served by some community-based mental health professionals. These services have varied from the more extensive community mental health centres found in the United States and parts of Eastern Europe, to the community nursing outreach services that have developed in Britain. In keeping with the approach we have advocated throughout, it is considered important to examine the relative merits of the existing services to the community, and to build on their strengths. For this reason we would suggest that allocation of resources should focus on supporting existing competent services in the community and integrating them into a coordinated service that meets the needs of the community in the most efficient manner. Where community-based resources already meet existing needs in an optimal manner, including facilitating the efficient reduction of impairment, disability and handicap associated with mental disorders, additional resources should be utilised to coordinate access to these resources and to support these efforts so that their standards are maintained. This allows scarce specialised resources to be devoted to areas where the existing community network has major deficiencies. Thus, where informal carers, family practitioners, employment programmes, day centres and housing agencies are coping with people with mental disorders without major difficulties, we would aim to support these services, providing consultation and training where indicated. In situations where such resources are unable to manage aspects of a case, we would expect the specialised mental health service to provide expert assistance with maximal efficiency. Where expertise for a particularly difficult problem was not available from the service, consultation would be arranged with services with the appropriate skills. This may include specialised medical, psychological or social agencies.

It is concluded that the existing network of resources, consisting mainly of the patients and their families – assisted by their family doctors, community nurses and social workers – are able to manage between 90 and 95% of all cases of mental disorders in the community. It is also evident that few family members or family doctors wish to have care of the people with mental disorders removed entirely from their jurisdiction. Most state a clear preference that they continue their roles as case managers, but are eager to share aspects of the care that are beyond their competence with expert mental health professionals. Almost all are keen to acquire a better understanding of mental disorders and effective treatment methods. Some groups of professionals such as the social workers and community nurses have expressed considerable interest in becoming more involved in the clinical management of persons with mental disorders. Other community agencies, such as the police and religious groups, complain that their training in dealing with persons with disabling mental disorders is grossly inadequate, yet they are often the first agencies contacted at times of crisis, and would welcome becoming part of an integrated service within the community.

In developing specialist mental health services, it is considered crucial that existing community resources are not disrupted, and that new services aim to support, rather than replace all care that is being provided in a competent manner.

Consultation must always remain a two-way process, and it is clear that the mental health professionals have as much to learn from the community caregivers as they have to offer in terms of specialist knowledge and skills. It seems essential to form an effective partnership, not merely with the primary care professionals, but above all with the patients and their caregivers, who represent the greatest resource for any community-based service. Integration with the existing community services might enable the 5 to 10% of persons not managed effectively under the current organisation to be treated successfully. In this way a relatively small specialist service may have a major impact on the large number of persons with mental disorders in the community.

Implementing integrated mental health services

Implementing a community-based mental health service that integrates all existing resources to ensure optimal resolution of the comprehensive mental health needs of the community requires careful planning. This task is much easier where needs and goals have been carefully assessed and resources targeted to those areas where they may achieve maximum efficiency. However, the detailed strategies that are employed are crucial. These should include methods to ensure that informal, primary and specialist resources are fully integrated, accessibility and acceptability maintained, and perhaps of greatest importance, that the most effective treatment is provided for every case.

The precise strategies used in the organisation of any service will depend on local factors. However, some general principles will apply to all services. Table 1.3 lists key strategies used in a service that was developed in a community that was well served by competent primary care services. In this instance family practitioners provided a comprehensive 24-hour service seven days a week. The population was fairly stable, with the result that people changed their doctor rarely, and families were usually registered with the same doctor. In such circumstances it made good sense to preserve the role of the

Table 1.3. *Strategies used in integrated services*

Family practitioner manager continuously
No waiting lists; no clinics; appointments mutual
24-hour intensive clinical management
Home-based management; carer always involved
Only mental disorders treated, including prodromes
Biopsychosocial management of every case
Least restrictive treatment strategies
Focus staff training on effective strategies only
Clinical decision making a scientific process

family doctor as the case manager throughout. All consultations with the specialist mental health professionals were made through the family doctor, including those from social and community agencies or other medical specialists. Several family doctors had high levels of competence in the clinical management of some mental disorders, others had very limited competence. In order to integrate the specialist and primary mental health services a shared care approach was developed. Small multidisciplinary teams of mental health professionals were allocated to each family practice group. They were provided with offices adjacent to the family doctors and community nurses. The specialist service was organised in a manner that mirrored the primary care service, with specialist consultation, including domiciliary assessment and treatment provided on a 24-hour basis, minimal formality associated with the consultation process, shared record keeping, and home-based management of episodes of major disorders that included all informal carers in the assessment and treatment process. Each mental health professional in the team shared care of a number of cases with each family practitioner. He or she organised other professionals within the team, as well as other resources in the community to ensure that the optimal management was provided to each case on a continuing basis.

It is clear that this type of service could not be established in communities where family practice was poorly developed, or where 24-hour care was not provided by the primary care team. However, one aspect of the service that would not change despite differing organisational structures would be the focus on effective clinical management strategies. The most important aspect of developing effective and efficient mental health services is having a well-trained staff team. Too often it is assumed that well-trained professionals ensure that they continue their professional development so that they remain highly competent in the latest technical skills associated with their discipline. Unfortunately, with few incentives to keep abreast of new developments, or to pursue often quite arduous training courses, relatively few mental health professionals are able to provide effective assessment and treatment strategies. Furthermore, left to their own devices, and the vagaries of the marketplace, even conscientious professionals will pursue training that may not be in accord with objective criteria for effective and efficient strategies. This may mean that a group of professionals will acquire a rag bag of skills, underpinned by contrasting theories, which may be incompatible in practice. Thus, careful planning of shared training in assessment and intervention procedures may lead to substantial enhancement of clinical efficacy as well as efficient team work. Wherever possible this training should be conducted in a multidisciplinary fashion. It is crucial that training extends to all members of the primary care service, who are all trained in methods of screening for major mental disorders.

The choice of effective therapeutic strategies has been facilitated by recent research that has established the efficacy of specific interventions for most of the major mental disorders (see Chapter 3). In most cases a biopsychosocial approach that integrates judicious use of drug and biological treatments with psychosocial strategies produces the optimal results. Training should be restricted to those strategies that have been demonstrated as most effective in the resolution of common mental disorders in rigorous, replicated controlled trials. Where two or more strategies have been demonstrated as having equal benefits, the choice should be based upon the cost of applying each strategy. Costs should involve the direct costs associated with the strategy as well as the costs of training and maintaining professional competence in the approach, and the risks of harmful effects, including restrictions placed upon an individual's freedom of choice associated with administration of the procedure. Treatments that lack scientific validation of their effectiveness should have no place in modern mental health services. Nor indeed, should strategies that, although effective, have been superseded by more potent or more efficient methods. Decisions about the choice of strategies to form the basis for the service must be made on a purely scientific basis, free of ideological or philosophical considerations apart from those associated with professional ethics. For problems where no specific interventions have been demonstrated effective, the scientific approach may be applied within a single-case design. A specific therapeutic goal is set, a specific intervention approach agreed, and the results measured systematically so that the merits of the approach can be evaluated. Such structure tends to facilitate optimal clinical management, providing specific feedback to sufferers, carers and professionals alike. Within such an approach a wide range of creative strategies may be refined that may lead to further therapeutic advances.

The manner in which service training is organised has not been subjected to extensive research. However, it is unlikely that any one approach will meet the various needs of a multidisciplinary staff of varying levels of expertise. However, it seems crucial that sufficient time and funds are allocated to ensure that all staff are trained to a high level of competence in the skills they need to meet the needs of the community in an efficient manner. Ideally this training should be provided prior to opening the service, with new members receiving extensive preparation before they begin duties within the teams. Until staff have met clear criteria for competence in the assessment and treatment of specific cases, they should not be permitted to carry out such procedures, except under the strictest supervision from a qualified member of the service.

Reviewing the progress of case management

In order to assess whether clinical practice is being implemented in the most effective and efficient manner it is essential to measure the progress of treatment. With a wide range of strategies being applied to a wide range of problems by a wide range of therapists, this presents some major difficulties. Two forms of assessment are needed. The first, to assess progress on the idiosyncratic problems presented by each case. The second, to compare the levels of impairment, disability and handicap between cases. In addition, it may help to record background information, diagnosis, problem assessment, management plans, and progress notes in a systematic fashion for all cases.

Progress on the specific problems and goals of each case that are targeted for intervention may be measured in idiosyncratic scales that are appropriate to each problem or goal. A wide range of such methods have been devised. These include measuring the frequency that a specific event occurs (e.g. panic attack, hallucination, performance of a social skill, etc.); or estimating the severity of a specific phenomenon on a linear rating scale (e.g. level of anxiety, urge to commit suicide, belief in a delusional thought). These ratings are specific to each individual and are devised so that they provide an accurate reflection of change in the problems specified in that person's management plan. They are conducted at regular intervals by the therapist in charge of the case. The patterns of change enable modifications of the course of an intervention program to be made according to the ratings that are observed. Presentation of this data forms a crucial aspect of the case review process within the multidisciplinary teams.

Standardised ratings of impairment, disability and handicap enable comparisons between cases with markedly different presenting problems. We would advocate the use of straightforward global ratings that can be readily applied at frequent intervals in the clinical setting, rather than more elaborate interviews and questionnaires that require extensive training of raters to achieve adequate levels of reliability in their application. The latter assessments are more useful in surveys that may be undertaken at less frequent intervals.

Systematic recording of background data on cases may form the basis for a computerised register of cases. This may be used in reviews of the outcome of the service as a whole; for monitoring long-term case management; and for developing a register of people considered to have a high risk of developing episodes of major mental disorders in the future.

The use of standardised assessments of progress are of little use unless mental health professionals are trained to make reliable ratings on the various scales chosen by the service. Regular recalibration with expert raters should be planned to maintain good inter-rater agreement.

Outcome assessment of the costs and benefits of the service

The last aspect in planning a comprehensive mental health service that addresses the specific needs of a community entails developing a method of providing feedback on all aspects of service delivery. These indicators of the strengths and weaknesses should reflect accurately the efficiency of the service in achieving the specific goals set for a defined period, usually one year. The focus should be on the *quality* of the therapeutic efficiency of the interventions provided rather than on measures such as numbers of consultations, or the case loads of therapists. Records of levels of impairment, disability and handicap, including that suffered by informal carers provide a more accurate reflection of the benefits achieved by the service, as well as evidence of areas where needs are not being met in an optimal fashion. In addition, these quantitative measures of benefit must be considered in terms of the costs involved in their achievement. Fiscal costs of a community-based service comprise mainly staff salaries, to which are added ancillary services of other community agencies, such as social services, the primary care resources, police assistance and hospital or other residential care. The added costs of informal carers, who may have to take unpaid leave from their jobs should be included. Emotional burdens of carers should not be neglected, but these are estimated in the levels of disability and handicap experienced by these crucial assistants. Ideally, publicly funded services should attempt to achieve maximum benefits with minimal costs. However, a few complicated cases with high levels of disability and handicap may require substantial staff resources, merely to prevent further deterioration. In order to improve the benefit/cost ratio it may be tempting to reduce the therapeutic input to persons with unrewarding conditions, and to seek out less complex cases that benefit more readily. While it is crucial to review these cases thoroughly in order to refine the therapeutic efforts that they are receiving, it is equally important that those with the highest needs are apportioned the most intensive and extensive clinical management, especially as new therapeutic advances enable more and more previously intractable disorders to be treated. Nevertheless, by enhancing the efficiency in the management of more straightforward cases, more time and effort can be devoted to resolving the difficulties of these refractory cases.

Comprehensive annual audits that examine the quality of the service provided as well as its efficiency in achieving specific goals allows detection of both the successes as well as the emerging problems. If the needs of the community are being met this should be reflected in a lowering of the prevalence of severe levels of impairment, disability and handicap in both sufferers and carers. Improved accessibility and acceptability of case management should lead to increased numbers of persons seeking help at progressively earlier stages in their disorders. Efficient management with effective therapeutic strategies may reduce their risk of developing severe disability and handicaps. Surveys of current consumers as well as potential consumers in the community may provide evidence of satisfaction and public attitudes towards the service, and suggest changes that might further enhance the ability of the service to meet the mental health needs of all people in the community.

References

Dilling H. & Weyerer S. (1984) Prevalence of mental disorders in the small town rural region of Traunstein (Upper Bavaria). *Acta Psychiatrica Scandinavica*, **69**, 60–79.

Faris R.E.L. & Dunham H.W. (1939) *Mental disorders in urban areas.* University of Chicago Press, Chicago.

Goldberg D.P. & Bridges K. (1987) Screening for psychiatric illness in general practice. *Journal of the Royal College of General Practitioners*, **37**, 15–19.

Goldberg D.P. & Huxley P. (1980) *Mental illness in the community.* Tavistock Press, London.

Guy W. (1976) *E.C.D.E.U. assessment manual for psychopharmacology.* U.S. Department of Health, Education and Welfare, Washington D.C.

Hafner H. & Reimann H. (1970) Spatial distribution of mental disorders in Mannheim, 1965. In E.H. Hare & J.K. Wing (eds) *Psychiatric Epidemiology.* Oxford University Press, Oxford, pp 341–354.

Lamb H.R. & Goertzel V. (1970) Discharged mental patients – are they really in the community? *Archives of General Psychiatry*, **24**, 29–34.

Lamb H.R. & Zusman J. (1981) A new look at primary prevention. *Hospital and Community Psychiatry*, **12**, 843–848.

Parkes C.M. (1978) On the use of psychiatric resources for indirect service. *Bulletin, Royal College of Psychiatrists*, 29–33.

Raeburn J.M. & Seymour F.W. (1977) Planning and evaluating community health and related projects: a systems approach. *New Zealand Medical Journal*, **86**, 188–190. p188.

Regier D.A., Burke J.D., Manderscheid R.W. & Burns B.J. (1985) The chronically mentally ill in primary care. *Psychological Medicine*, **15**, 265–273.

Regier D.A., Myers J.K. Kramer M., Robins L.N., Blazer D.G., Hough R.L., Eaton W.W. & Locke B.Z. (1984) The NIMH Epidemiological Catchment Area program: Historical context, major objectives and study population characteristics. *Archives of General Psychiatry*, **41**, 934–941.

Sartorius N., Jablensky A. & Shapiro R. (1977) Two year-follow-up of the patients included in the WHO International Pilot Study of Schizophrenia. *Psychological Medicine*, **7**, 529–541.

Shepherd M., Cooper B., Brown A.C. & Kalton G. (1966) *Psychiatric illness in general practice*. Oxford University Press, Oxford.

Warner R. (1985) *Recovery from schizophrenia*. Routledge & Kegan Paul, London.

Wing J.K. (1968) Social treatments of mental illness. In M. Shepherd & D.L.Davies (eds) *Studies in psychiatry*. Oxford University Press, Oxford.

Wing J.K., Cooper J.E. & Sartorius N. (1974) *The measurement and classification of psychiatric symptoms*. Cambridge University Press, London.

2

Community management of mental disorders: integrating patients, carers, primary health care with specialist mental health services

Introduction. Vulnerability–stress: a model for intervention

In order to ensure that each person in a community who is suffering impairments, disabilities or handicaps associated with mental disorders receives the optimal combination of effective biopsychosocial interventions it may be useful to adopt a rationale for the pathogenesis of mental disorders that is shared by most of the common disorders and can provide a guideline to therapists who are attempting to assess and treat cases on a long-term need-related basis. The vulnerability–stress model is one generic approach that we have considered useful as a basis for clinical management of most cases. We have derived this model from the seminal work of George Brown and his colleagues at the Medical Research Council's Social Psychiatry Unit, and more recently, the Sociology Department of Bedford College, London.

The vulnerability–stress model of mental disorders postulates that the impairment of mental disorders is most likely to become manifest at times when the combination of vulnerability and stress factors overwhelms an individual's biopsychosocial adjustment capacity and triggers off the biobehavioural responses that characterise that person's disorder (see Figure 2.1). *Vulnerability* refers to factors that predispose a person to develop a particular syndrome at any point in time. Relatively little is currently known about the specific factors that contribute to specific mental disorders. Genetic predisposition has been found in most major mental disorders. The preexistence of a mental disorder in a first degree relative (i.e. parent or sibling) tends to increase the risk of developing a similar mental

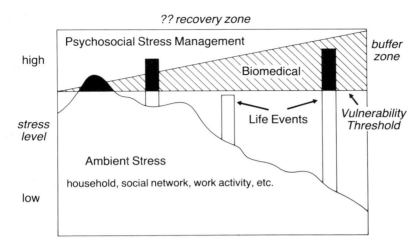

Figure 2.1. The vulnerability–stress model of mental disorders.

disorder significantly above that of the general population. However, in most cases the increased risk is not substantial, and the patterns of genetic transmission remain unclear. Higher inherited risk appears in persons where an identical twin suffers a disorder, or where both parents have had a disorder. A few families have been found where unusually high rates of specific disorders have been observed. Such families have excited great enthusiasm among researchers seeking specific genetic deficits for schizophrenia and manic-depressive conditions. However, such research remains inconclusive at present, and has yet to lead to the detection of any biomedical or psychosocial markers of those family members who might be most prone to the disorder before they become impaired. Nevertheless, it seems clear that inherited factors account for at least some of the vulnerability to mental disorders, and that any person with a first degree member of their family who has experienced a major mental disorder should be considered to have a higher risk of developing some form of mental disorder than others in the general population.

It may be presumed that genetic vulnerability is mediated through some abnormalities in brain metabolism, and that it is this weakness that contributes to the development of the disorder under certain conditions. Biochemical research has uncovered a large number of such abnormalities in persons with established mental disorders. Abnormalities in the metabolism of dopamine have been associated with schizophrenic disorders, and abnormalities of thyroid and adrenal hormones have been associated with affective disorders. Once again, no specific hypotheses have to date clearly linked specific abnormalities to patterns of impairment. Biochemical research is extraordinarily difficult to control, with factors such as nutritional status and physical activity potentially confounding results. Nevertheless, every mental activity is associated with biochemical responses of neurotransmitters in the brain, so it is reasonable to assume that mental disorders and biochemical abnormalities are inextricably linked.

However, those links are seldom straightforward relationships. For example, some persons who suffer panic disorders have a tendency to hyperventilate, this tendency is enhanced by stress and tension; the odd sensations created by the biochemical changes induced by hyperventilation are then interpreted as threatening, even life threatening (e.g. as having a heart attack or stroke), and contribute to the overwhelming anxiety experienced by the sufferer. Thus, biochemical changes are not always sufficient to cause mental disorders on their own, but may require the interaction with psychological and social factors to produce disabling disorders. Psychological traits that determine individuals' cognitive appraisal patterns may determine whether a biochemical change is interpreted in a positive, negative or neutral fashion, and results in further escalation of the mood disturbance, or is passed off as a merely discomforting sensation. The physiological changes in the female hormones during the menstrual cycle, throughout pregnancy and childbirth, and at the menopause lead to a wide range of response patterns, that contribute to the varying vulnerability associated with such changes.

Pre-existing brain dysfunction, such as that associated with birth injury, viral encephalitis or epilepsy, appears to be another factor that enhances the vulnerability to major mental disorders including schizophrenia (Lewis & Murray, 1987).

Environmental stress is postulated as playing a role in triggering episodes of impairment in persons who are otherwise predisposed to a specific disorder. The risk of experiencing an episode appears to be increased where stress exceeds an individual's vulnerability threshold. The level of this threshold is determined by a person's overall vulnerability at any point in time. Exceeding this threshold will tend to trigger physiological and psychological stress responses and is associated with a high risk of impaired health. Two types of stressor have been researched: ambient stress and life events.

Ambient stress is the stress experienced in dealing with the day-to-day hassles of life in the community. It is an accumulation of stresses in the household, social and leisure pursuits, and in work activities. Stressors covering such a wide range are extremely difficult to quantify. However, household stress has been measured by indices such as 'expressed emotion' (Vaughn & Leff, 1976) and 'family burden' (Grad & Sainsbury, 1963). Work-related stress and stress in social relationships, including the stresses associated with home-making, childcare, unemployment, and interpersonal relationships have been less readily measured, yet are undoubtedly as important as family relationships as sources of ambient stress. Indices of household stress have predicted the risk of recurrent episodes of schizophrenic and affective disorders (Leff and Vaughn, 1985; Miklowitz et al, 1988). Persisting high levels of ambient stress in the environment have similarly predicted the development of depressive disorders (Brown & Harris, 1978).

A life event is the term used to define more discrete stresses, such as the loss of a job, death of a close associate or break-up of an intimate relationship. Life events that lead to long-term ambient stress have been associated with the onset of major episodes of depressive (Brown & Harris, 1978), schizophrenic (Brown & Birley 1968), manic (Ambelas, 1987), and anxiety disorders (Tennant & Andrews, 1978). The mechanisms for the pathogenic effects of such stresses have not been clearly delineated.

However, it is evident that it is each person's subjective appraisal of the threatening impact of any event, coupled with their perceived ability to cope with the associated stress that is most closely associated with the onset of impairment. We postulate that such cognitive awareness of stress is often associated with physiological change in vulnerable biological pathways, thereby contributing to episodes of impairment. Relatively little research has been conducted to support this hypothesis, but there is some evidence for increased physiological arousal associated with environmental stress in schizophrenia (Tarrier et al, 1979).

It has been noted that there is substantial variation in the patterns of physiological change (including biochemical responses) observed

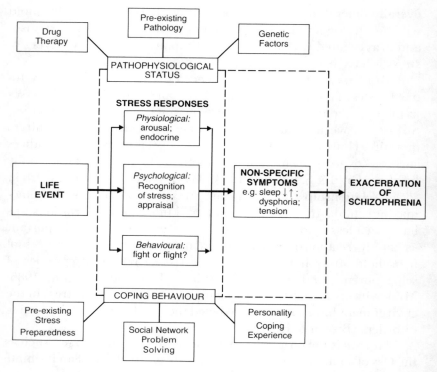

Figure 2.2. The role of life events, coping mechanisms and prophylactic interventions in episodes of schizophrenia.

in individual cases, even within a group of people experiencing the same mental disorders. Similar variation in the cognitive and behavioural responses to stresses have been found. It is likely that a person's response to stress is multidetermined, with biogenetic factors determining physiological response patterns, and psychological factors, such as personality, conditioning to past experiences, coping skills and being prepared for an expected occurrence, all determining the individual's actions in response to the specific stress. The multiplicity of factors that determine the stress responses of a person who is vulnerable to schizophrenic episodes is summarised in Figure 2.2. This may appear substantially more complex than many simple cause–effect relationships postulated by advocates of single-factor origins for specific mental disorders. But it is substantially less complex than the current understanding of the control of the circulatory system (Figure 2.3), which is a relatively simple engineering feat, and undoubtedly less complex than any mechanism controlling central nervous system functions. The reader, therefore, should be cautioned against believing that any of our simplistic models of mental dysfunctions are anything more than reflections of the highly primitive understanding we have of the precise mechanisms that operate. Nevertheless, such simple models may prove helpful in guiding our therapeutic efforts in a manner that facilitates integration of the best strategies we have at our disposal currently.

Stress does not interact in a direct manner with vulnerability to produce the specific impairments that characterise specific mental disorders. It appears that stress responses may lead to a range of impairments in any individual. Although the possibilities are extensive, most persons have a more restricted range of non-specific impairments that are characteristic stress responses for them. These impairments result from the excessive physiological changes that stress induces for that particular person. For example, one person experiences an increase in muscular tone that may lead to tension headaches or backache, another may have stress-induced increase in gastric acid leading to reduced appetite and indigestion, another may have an increase in adrenergic activity leading to difficulty relaxing and disturbed sleep patterns. In persons vulnerable to specific mental disorders these impairments may precede the onset of the specific features of the disorders to which they are especially prone, such as perceptual disturbances, mood changes, or behavioural abnormalities. The ability to recognise the prodromal nature of specific effects of stress, may assist the person to seek early intervention and help modify the course of major episodes of mental disorders. The definition of these non-specific early warning signs may facilitate efficient crisis intervention aimed at buffering and subsequently resolving persisting stress, as well as countering the physiological responses with drugs or other agents to alter the biological patterns; these may include hormonal adjustment to reduce premenstrual vulnerability or relaxation to modify muscle tension.

The indirect mediation of stress responses usually means that there is a delay between the onset of an overwhelming stressor and the development of an episode of a mental disorder. This delay may be a matter of hours in the case of persons with pre-existing impairments (i.e. persisting subacute symptoms of a mental disorder), or extend over several months in the case of some depressive

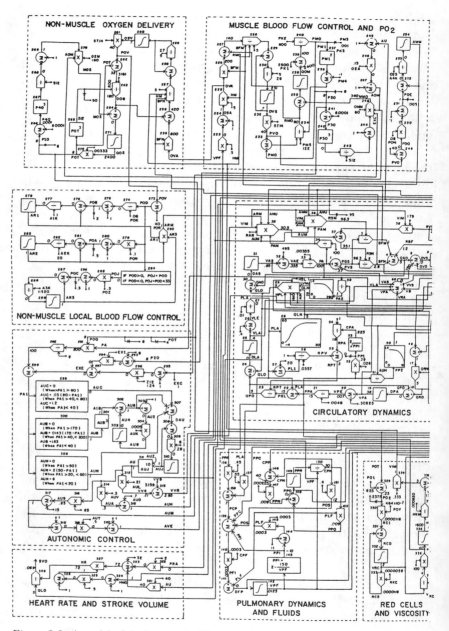

Figure 2.3. A model of the human circulatory system.

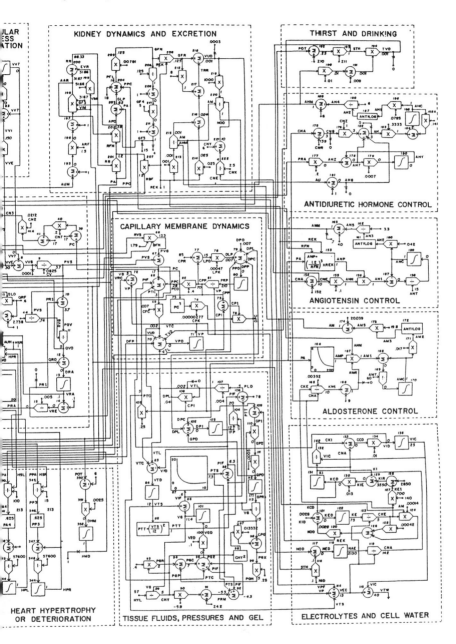

episodes (Brown & Harris, 1978). For most schizophrenic, anxiety and manic disorders the lag period between the onset of stress and the development of a major episode is several days. During this time prodromal signs will be evident, and crisis intervention may avert a major episode or at least modify its severity.

Implications of the vulnerability–stress model for mental health services

Several principles for the delivery of mental health services may be derived from the vulnerability–stress model. These include:

(*a*) The need to screen people who have high levels of vulnerability to mental disorders, and to ensure that they receive competent early mental health assessment when they show early signs of possible mental disorders.

(*b*) A longitudinal perspective for persons who develop mental disorders that ensures that any reversible vulnerability factors are treated, that clinical management is continuous, with efforts directed at efficient stress management by optimal combinations of biological, psychological and social procedures. These will vary according to the specific needs of each individual at each phase of their disorder.*

(*c*) A teamwork approach to case management that integrates medical, nursing, psychological, occupational and social assessments and effective treatment strategies with the long-term goal of

---

* *Stress management* is frequently equated with *stress reduction*. However, we believe that the distinction is very important. Stress management is the capacity of an individual to cope with the stresses they encounter, and involves the ability to assess current and potential stressors, gauge their likely effects, plan and carry out effective strategies to efficiently resolve high stress levels before they exceed that person's threshold, and threaten his or her health status. Stress reduction is one type of strategy that a person may employ to manage stress at any time. It is particularly useful at times when stress overwhelms a person's coping capacity, when combinations of tranquillising drugs and withdrawal from the stresses of everyday social roles may assist in the rapid reduction of severe stress. However, such methods that have dramatic short-term benefits tend to have major disadvantages when employed on a longer-term basis, as has been evidenced by the unwanted effects of many drug regimens, as well as by those of extensive avoidance and escape strategies characterised by asylums – both those provided by institutional care, particularly for those vulnerable to schizophrenic episodes, as well as asylums created at home, of the kinds created by many carers of people prone to anxiety and depressive disorders.

   Effective stress management aims at assisting all vulnerable persons to lead unrestricted lives through learning to cope with higher levels of environmental stress in a more effective and efficient manner. This learning is seen as a lifelong process that few highly vulnerable people can ever abandon, without increasing their risk of deterioration in their health or well-being.

full recovery of community functioning, and above all ensures that the stress associated with the clinical management of mental disorders is minimised at all times.

(*d*) A locus of case management that facilitates an understanding of the vulnerability-stress model and its application in a highly consistent manner by patients, carers, and all professional therapists.

(*e*) The carers of people who are disabled by mental disorders are themselves often placed under considerable stress by their caregiving roles. In addition they often have increased vulnerability to mental disorders as a result of being first degree relatives, or assortative pairing (e.g. disabled persons sharing a household or marrying). Thus, clinical management should encompass both the index patient and the carers throughout.

(*f*) The need to extend stress management beyond the immediate household environment so that highly vulnerable people can learn to manage a full range of stresses in areas such as occupation, recreation, and intimate relations in a wider social network.

Models of comprehensive mental health services

The development of models of comprehensive mental health services based upon the vulnerability–stress hypothesis has occurred over the past 30 years. These models have evolved in parallel with developments in the clinical applications of the vulnerability–stress hypothesis. We have chosen to illustrate this evolutionary process by providing three examples of comprehensive services that have been considered at the forefront of developments during each of the last three decades. These are: (1) the hospital-based community mental health service; (2) the community-based approach; and (3) the integrated approach. The contrasting aspects of each are highlighted, as well as the manner in which each approach has built upon the strengths of the earlier model.

The hospital-based model

This approach has characterised most European developments in comprehensive mental health services, as well as the community mental health centres of the United States. It was initiated in the late

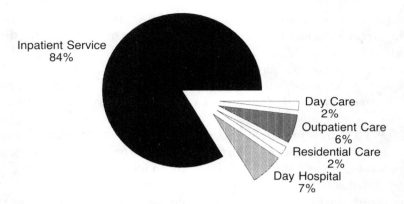

Figure 2.4. Expenditure on mental health services in England 1986/7: proportions of the total. (From Mental Health in the 1990s. *Office of Health Economics, 1989.)*

Table 2.1. *Resources for a hospital-based service (per 100,000 population)*

Inpatient beds	50
Day hospital places	25
Hostel/ward beds for 'new' long-stay	17
Short-term and rehabilitation hostels	4–6
Long-stay specialised accommodation	15–24
Day centre places	60

1960s and early 1970s. The key element of the service is considered the hospital inpatient service or its non-institutional equivalent, with supplementary outreach services to support patients once they have been discharged from the hospital (see Figure 2.4). The hospital is considered the locus for acute care as well as rehabilitation, with discharge secured when all impairment and disability has been minimised. Follow-up in the community setting has aimed to provide support to sustain the benefits achieved through the intensive treatment in the hospital setting. The main components of this service approach are summarised in Table 2.1. It is evident that the main focus is on the number of 'beds' required in a variety of settings.

Inpatient services

It can be seen that the major therapeutic input of such a service is provided by an inpatient unit, that focusses on crisis management of persons at the times that they are acutely disturbed. Although some effort has been made to devolve intensive crisis management from 24-hour care to less extensive day hospital care, the latter services are usually found at the same location as the inpatient unit. Efforts to make mental health care more accessible have led to the development of inpatient units in general hospitals or to attempts to apply therapeutic community methods. However, there is little evidence that either of these moves has enhanced the effectiveness or efficiency of crisis management.

Clinical management in inpatient units provides assessment of impairment in a structured, highly stressful environment, with closely monitored drug interventions. Easy accessibility to the facilities of a general hospital enables a range of biomedical investigations to be conducted and improves liaison with other medical specialists for those cases where collaborative management may be beneficial.

Other benefits that are claimed include the suggestion that people expressing suicidal or homicidal ideas are safer within an inpatient unit than in alternative community supervision. There is little evidence that hospitals provide any greater degree of safety than other settings in the community. However, in the case of violent behaviour, the targets of assaults are likely to be nursing staff and fellow sufferers, rather than carers and the general public.

Disadvantages of inpatient services include the difficulty of generalising assessments and treatment interventions to the person's natural living environment (Liberman et al, 1975). Typical examples of these problems are the assessment of a secretary's work skills in an industrial workshop, or the ability of a person to replicate tablet ingestion in the highly regulated manner of the hospital. Bennett (1982) pointed out the unsatisfactory nature of inpatient assessment of disability:

> If we are interested in assessing the role behaviour of a patient that behaviour can only be assessed by observing the person in a realistic

situation; it may be a work situation, a family situation or a social situation. It is quite clear that observation in the ward of a traditional hospital is not satisfactory. Nor is it adequate to make an assessment using tests, questionnaires or structured interviews. Real life situations can be introduced into hospital though this is rarely done.

Much has been made of the stigma associated with admission to a mental hospital. However, similar stigma is evident in other community settings and is more likely to be associated with mental disorders than the settings in which they are treated. Efforts to reduce the stigma associated with mental hospitals have taken contrasting directions. Initially, efforts to establish therapeutic communities aimed at breaking down the medical/nursing hierarchy, and creating a social system that resembled that of the ideal democratic socialist community. Such environments may have appeared to resemble community life more accurately, and gave more responsibility to patients. Unfortunately, they did not provide any additional therapeutic potential, and may have even reduced the therapeutic potency in the clinical management of some major disorders (May, 1968). A more recent development has resulted in attempts to make inpatient units for mental disorders resemble those for other medical conditions. This approach has yet to be evaluated, but it is doubtful that the case can be successfully argued that modern management of mental disorders should be focussed so extensively on the biomedical aspects of management. Donald Dick (1982) offered an excellent description of the role of the inpatient service:

> The function of the bed in psychiatry differs from the function of the bed in other branches of medicine. It is usually the place where the patient sleeps at night during a period of treatment or observation. It is not as important as the treatment place although it clearly has an essential role in assessment, observation, investigation, necessary separation and, at times of acute illness, containment. However, the majority of psychiatrically troubled people are best sleeping in their own beds at night, holding their place in their own surroundings and family structure and not in exile.

Day hospitals

One attempt to reduce dependence on large numbers of inpatient beds that has been advocated for hospital-based services is the day hospital. The aim of day hospitals is to provide all the resources of an inpatient unit from 9 a.m. to 5 p.m. during weekdays for acutely disturbed people, who return to their informal carers overnight and for weekends and holidays. A few services have identified a separate need for a night hospital, particularly for persons attending day hospitals or work programmes in the community who require supported lodgings before they are able to cope with both working and living independently (Harris, 1957; Gudeman and Shore, 1984).

There are no studies to indicate whether day hospitals improve the accessibility of care to the community, even when they have been sited outside the confines of hospital grounds. However, the results of intensive care provided in this manner suggests that they may provide an effective alternative to inpatient management for a high proportion of cases, at least reducing the length of inpatient stay and facilitating early discharge (Creed et al, 1989).

The specific intervention provided in day treatment programmes is poorly standardised and varies considerably. Effectiveness appears greatest where the focus of treatment is on each person's living skills, including self care, social skills and work activity; and where these skills are taught using individualised behavioural methods in addition to optimal drug therapy, rather than those based upon milieu, group or psychodynamic methods (Austin et al, 1976; Linn et al, 1979; Falloon & Talbot, 1982).

Day care

Day care services are frequently confused with day hospitals. Their goals are to provide support for people with long-term disability who are considered unable to work or to utilise the range of non-specialised recreational and leisure resources that exist in the community. They may be considered an attempt to replicate the sheltered social environments provided in the traditional mental hospitals. There is no evaluation of the effectiveness of such programmes in reducing disability or handicaps associated with major mental disorders.

Sheltered workshops, particularly those with low expectancy of progress towards open employment, may be considered a specialised form of day care. Their focus on industrial-type work has tended to limit their clientele. Recent developments have included the development of small community businesses staffed by clients and volunteers. Ventures, such as coffee shops or restaurants, offer a broad range of jobs that enable people with different levels of disability to function in a productive and satisfying manner.

Outpatient clinics

The hospital-based outpatient clinic is a major component of these community services. It combines a number of functions:

1 Screening for mental disorders
2 Clinical management of established mental disorders where disturbed behaviour that frequently leads to rejection by community carers is not a major issue.
3 Psychosocial crisis intervention for distressed persons who do not have mental disorders but have similar levels of disability in their interpersonal relationships and social role functioning in the community. In many programs this may extend indefinitely, involving multiple crises.
4 Clinical management of maintenance medication for persons after hospital discharge.
5 Outreach domiciliary nursing and crisis management of disabled persons.

Outpatient services provide a crucial link between the hospital and the community. They form a major component of most community mental health clinics where clinical management is provided by professionals from all disciplines. The manner in which the various disciplines work together varies from the team approach where all disciplines manage cases in a standardised biopsychosocial way, to a series of specialised clinics run by each discipline. Little research has been conducted to establish the relative merits of these two approaches, although at least one study has found little difference in outcome between cases managed by nurses and those managed by psychiatrists (Paykel et al, 1982).

Among the disadvantages of traditional outpatient units are that they are often, staffed by trainees, who change frequently, thereby reducing continuity of care; attendance rates are poor, with little follow-up of non-attenders; and usually only the patient is assessed, with limited assessment of the carers and social stressors.

Delivery of traditional services has been modified in a number of ways to enhance accessibility and acceptability. These include: the provision of walk-in consultation that obviates the often lengthy waits for appointments; clinics provided in town centres, housing developments and family practices; home-based provision of drug treatment; and home-based psychiatric assessment of crises. Such innovations have undoubtedly assisted in the early detection of major episodes of mental disorders, as well as assisting primary and informal caregivers in their case management roles.

Home-based drug treatment provided primarily by skilled nurses has been evaluated by Pasamanick and his colleagues (1967). This study suggested that long-term drug treatment for persons recovering from schizophrenic episodes could be successfully managed by teams of nurses supported by psychiatrists, who assisted in the maintenance of compliance, assessed side effects, and monitored the early signs of recurrences. This approach reduced the rate of hospital admissions when compared with the traditional outpatient services. It may be important to note that this project used oral neuroleptic drugs, and demonstrated that compliance could be maintained with a well organised programme that involved both patients and their informal carers.

The provision of specialised mental health consultation in family practice has been a recent development in the UK. Studies have revealed that at least 25% of consultant psychiatrists conduct some of their outpatient services in family practices (Strathdee & Williams, 1984). Nurses, social workers and psychologists have also begun to provide services within the primary care sector. Three controlled studies have examined the benefits of locating outpatient services in primary care facilities. Psychological treatment approaches have been shown to be more effective than routine family practice when provided either by psychologists or nurses trained in psychological treatment methods (Marks, 1985; Robson et al, 1984). Social workers proved no more effective than routine primary care in treating a sample of depressed women, although there was some evidence that their counselling approach was most beneficial with acute exacerbations of chronic disorders (Corney, 1981).

While these and other studies suggest that persons with interpersonal problems and mild to moderate anxiety disorders are more likely to attend consultations provided in the more accessible setting of primary care, there is no evidence that the more severely impaired take advantage of this change in the locus of care, and hospital admissions for these conditions probably remain the same (Williams & Balestrieri, 1989).

It is clear that outpatient services can be provided in home-based and primary care settings, and that this may provide a more accessible service for persons with mental disorders. However, such outreach services are generally organised by professional groups, isolated from other disciplines. Whereas in a traditional outpatient clinic such professional separation may be less critical, with psychiatry, nursing, psychology, social work and occupational therapy departments all in close proximity, the move out of an institutional base may lead to reduced interdisciplinary management.

Another drawback attributable to improved accessibility of outpatient care is highlighted by the fact that many persons appear to derive equal benefits from the treatments provided by primary care and mental health professionals. No method has yet been tested for discriminating between cases that the primary care team treats effectively and those who are likely to require more specialist intervention. Shepherd et al (1966) proposed that rather than take over the role of primary care, mental health services should first offer consultation to the primary care professionals so that they may enhance their skills in assessing and treating mental disorders. Close liaison such as that implemented by Mitchell (1983), is an excellent model of this approach that has been well received by family practitioners and their staff. Ideally, family practitioners' basic training should equip them with the skills to effectively screen cases of mental disorders and provide relatively straightforward treatment interventions for uncomplicated cases. However, most training programmes are conducted in inpatient units, and provide minimal guidance on the management of such cases.

The stigma associated with serious mental disorders remains a major block to persons seeking early treatment. One of the explicit goals of community-based mental health care was to provide public education about the nature of mental disorders and their management, in order to minimise stigma. Unfortunately, few effective programmes have been developed and even fewer have been evaluated. The integration of mental health services with family practice and the resultant increased involvement with family members would seem to offer an excellent opportunity to deliver mental health education to the community as a whole. Liaison with advocacy groups has led to the development of carer support groups and improvement in the education about mental disorders, at least for those carers who assist in the management of severely disabled people (McGill et al, 1983).

Residential alternatives to hospital

Hospital-based community services have attempted to reduce the expenditure on inpatient units by developing residential alternatives to the hospital ward. These vary from houses that essentially replicate the intensive clinical management provided in a hospital ward, but are located in a residential setting (Wykes & Wing, 1982; Mosher & Menn, 1978; Warner, 1985), to subsidised housing programmes.

There is limited evidence that the provision of intensive treatment of major episodes of mental disorders is more effective in residential style settings, or indeed any cheaper. However, it is probable that people with mental disorders prefer to be treated in homelike settings, and that admission of reluctant individuals may prove less coercive. Nevertheless, few households are equipped to cope with the stress of caring for *one* person experiencing a major episode of a mental disorder, and it is doubtful whether community wards are able to reduce environmental stress substantially for a group of disturbed people. The stress research has shown that it is the quality of interpersonal support that is crucial, not merely the physical surroundings. Excellent examples of these residential alternatives are well equipped with highly motivated staff, who display excellent skills in stress management, and are supported by specialist psychiatrists, psychologists and other experts who share their enthusiasm for the non-institutional approach (Mosher & Burti, 1989).

The stress of inadequate housing is a major contributor to recurring and persistent impairment associated with mental disorders. Moreover, the public misperception of persons who suffer mental disorders as threatening, undesirable citizens, handicaps them in the competition for access to housing resources in their communities. This problem is compounded where mental hospitals have admitted people as a direct consequence of their housing crises, as an expedient to assisting in resolving the housing problem in a direct manner. As a result mental hospitals have become a major part of the housing provided for communities, with a large proportion of their capacity utilised in this manner at any time. Closure

of such hospitals is only feasible where community housing programmes address this need in an adequate fashion, and where such
programmes do not discriminate against people who have had
mental disorders. A range of specialised housing is needed for
persons with disabilities. This includes the provision of a range of
supportive services to cope with individualised needs in a range of
settings. However, it is debatable whether health services should
become purveyors of housing themselves, or work with housing
agencies to provide appropriate resources that are compatible with
health maintenance and rehabilitation of all disabled people.

Staff training in hospital-based settings

The hospital-based model of community mental health care has
tended to provide training along single discipline lines. Each profession has adopted an apprenticeship model, supplemented by
lectures and seminars to train staff in the core skills of that discipline.
Case studies are conducted where trainees attempt to replicate the
clinical management their tutors have instructed them about, and
occasionally demonstrated for them. These studies are presented
orally, either in supervised discussion with the tutor, or in written
reports for more formal assessment.

Interdisciplinary training is encouraged, but the emphasis is more
on learning how the other specialist services work, including their
referral practices, rather than on training in the core skills associated
with those professional groups. In some instances restrictive practices have been developed by some professions to actively discourage
the sharing of profession skills with other disciplines within the
mental health field. Research into the most efficient and effective
methods of training staff is negligible, and attempts to evaluate the
continuing competence of professionals in their performance of
specific skills have not been validated. It is concluded that there is a
substantial need for a review of the training of professional staff to
provide comprehensive state-of-the-art mental health services that
meet the needs of all persons experiencing the impairments, disabilities and handicaps associated with mental disorders.

Community-based mental health services

The community-based approach to the delivery of mental health
services may seem similar to the hospital-based approach in many

ways. Many of the services are provided in a similar manner. However, the main distinction is that there is a strong emphasis on providing all services from a community base that is not a hospital. The basis for the service is considered to be ambulatory care service aimed at supporting people in their own social habitats throughout all phases of their disorders, with an emphasis on individualised interventions as an alternative to the centralised group treatment provided in hospital-based services. In other words, the hospital is seen as the last resort, and the least extensive component of the service, rather than the key resource from which all other programmes emanate.

Perhaps the best developed model of a community-based service is the Dane County service in Wisconsin, USA, that has evolved over the last 20 years, associated with the leadership of Mary Ann Test and Leonard Stein (Stein & Test, 1980; 1985). This programme has inspired many similar developments throughout the world, including Australia, Italy and more recently in the UK.

The key components of this approach are:

1 Community-based crisis intervention and intensive care.
2 Mobile community rehabilitation.
3 Supervised residential care.

These components are coordinated within an assertive team-based case management framework that ensures that all persons with major mental disorders in the community receive the clinical management that addresses their specific needs at each phase of their disorder.

Crisis intervention

This component of the service is the key entry point for most cases. People presenting in distressed states, who would be admitted to inpatient units in hospital-based approaches, are assessed on a 24-hour basis without delay. Assessment is conducted by a multidisciplinary team of highly skilled professionals, who aim to define the specific deficiencies in the needs of the individual and his social network support that appear to have contributed to the crisis. These needs are then met immediately with intensive social support and medication, as appropriate. The intensive intervention is applied in the community on a 24-hour basis, similar to that provided in an excellent inpatient unit. This may entail staff spending extended periods with the patient and his carers assisting with all aspects of daily living, such as food preparation, self-care, and occupational activity. This may include assistance in resolving major stresses, such as finding housing, or dealing with relationship difficulties. Although some efforts are made to teach the person more effective living skills this is generally done in a similar manner to hospital-based programs, with the therapist guiding the patient to perform the skills with assistance where needed. Explicit skill training for either patients or carers is not provided. However, this *in vivo* practice clearly avoids some of the problems associated with transfer of coping and living skills learned in a hospital setting into the natural environment.

Drugs are often administered by the professional team in a manner similar to that of the hospital ward. Where family carers are distressed, patients are usually removed from the household and cared for in less stressful residential settings in the community. These include low-stress hostels (Mosher & Menn, 1978) and foster homes (Polak & Kirby, 1976). In the latter, families are recruited in the community to provide short-term lodgings for patients in crisis, with the professional team assisting in providing specific inter-ventions. The families are paid for their services and are provided with training in the strategies that aim to reduce household stress during these periods of foster care.

It is apparent that this approach to crisis intervention provides all the resources of an excellent inpatient unit in a community setting. It is based mainly on psychosocial support and medication. The major advantages appear to be the manner in which patients are assisted to carry on their everyday roles in the community to the best of their ability and are helped to resolve stresses that are thought to have contributed to the current crisis. However, it is clear that this highly individualised approach is very labour-intensive and requires sub-stantial coordination among the members of the crisis team. Although research data suggests that around 80% of admissions to hospital can be avoided, there is relatively little evidence of added benefits in reductions in impairment, disability or handicap when this approach is compared with traditional inpatient crisis care (Stein & Test, 1980; Test & Stein, 1980; Fenton et al, 1981; Hoult, 1986). Surprisingly, one of the postulated drawbacks of such an approach, namely the added burden on informal carers, has not been observed. Where effective support is provided in this efficient needs-directed manner, carers experience less burden than when crisis care is undertaken in the hospital (Hoult, 1986).

Mobile community rehabilitation

The provision of continuing care to assist people to improve the quality of the lives and reduce residual impairments, disability and handicaps is a major concern of community-based mental health services that is shared with hospital-based approaches. However, whereas the hospital-based methods tend to favour centralising rehabilitation services in day hospitals, community wards, sheltered workshops and social day care programmes, the community-based approach favours a mobile programme that provides individually targeted interventions that account for the varying strengths and weaknesses of each person's living skills, and are provided in the person's natural habitat in the community. Participants are brought together into groups only when the group setting facilitates the intervention programme, such as to practice social skills, or to participate in group recreational activities.

Wherever possible participants are encouraged to integrate into existing programmes in the community, whether these involve leisure, recreation, work, education, housing or community service. Special efforts are made by professional case managers to facilitate access for the disabled into these community programmes. This includes continued assertive liaison with the business community, community leaders, all social, housing and educational agencies, and the local police services. The aim is to break down stigma and misunderstanding about the nature of mental disorders so that mentally disordered people are managed like any other member of the community. Acceptance of full citizen status, however, carries responsibility. Thus, persons suffering mental disorders or associated disability must accept the consequences of any misdemeanours or antisocial acts, in a manner similar to any citizen. This means that the label of mental disorder does not excuse the application of the legal processes of the community. Of course the levels of disability of an individual and their health status may determine the manner in which those legal constraints are employed, and in particular, the use of punishment (Stein & Diamond, 1985). With assertive liaison with the criminal justice system similar individualised programmes can be developed to ensure that law-breaking is minimised within the vulnerability–stress framework of each individual.

Long-term drug interventions are a major feature in the prevention of recurrent or persistent florid episodes of impairment for many people. The mobile rehabilitation model provides supervision of medication that ensures that adherence to the prescribed regimen is maintained. Community psychiatric nursing has played a major role in this crucial component of the service, particularly where neuroleptic drugs have been administered in depot injections. However, similar home-based supervision of tablet taking has been employed with similar success (Falloon et al, 1978). In addition to medication, prevention of florid episodes and social crises are achieved through supportive case management that aims to assist the person to achieve a stable lifestyle without excess stress. When unexpected stress occurs the community-based service ensures that professional support is provided to reduce the stress as efficiently as possible. In other words, both drugs and professional support are titrated to the vulnerable person's needs at any time.

It is assumed that such interventions may need to be provided for the most vulnerable people for the remainder of their lives. These people are not allowed to passively drop out from long-term care. They are closely monitored even when not receiving any active interventions, and considerable efforts are made to ensure that they find all key aspects of their treatment acceptable. In some circumstances this continuing care may be supported by compulsory court orders, such as guardianships, where professional case managers may adopt legal care to ensure that those vulnerable to developing disorders do not opt out of the monitoring process. In some places such compulsory orders may extend to the provision of community treatment. However, it is probable that most cases for whom compulsory treatment may be deemed beneficial can be managed without such coercive methods by assertive community-based teams, who usually advocate the use of the least restrictive approach.

The role of informal carers, particularly family members, is not always clearly defined in community-based care. In most programmes they are provided with education about the nature of mental disorders and the vulnerability–stress hypothesis, with the goal of assisting them to adopt low stress responses to irritating or upsetting behaviour that results from impairment and disability.

However, few programmes actively engage families in the rehabilitation programme, preferring to employ professional resources instead. A strong emphasis is often placed upon assisting the
vulnerable person to transfer his dependence from supportive family
members to supportive professional case managers, and to gain
'independence' from family carers. However, a major disadvantage
of this approach is the manner in which many vulnerable people
become excessively dependent on the unconditional support provided in the therapeutic relationship, especially where such dependence assists the therapy team to maintain close monitoring of these
cases. Under these circumstances even the temporary absence of a
person's case manager may be perceived as a major life event, and
the loss of such a person through job assignment changes may prove
catastrophic. Close professional teamwork may diffuse dependency
and ease potential stress. But as Richard Lamb has pointed out, the
same handicaps associated with long-term asylum in institutions are
readily replicated in community settings when similar practice is
replicated (Lamb & Goerzel, 1971; Lamb, 1979).

Supervised residential care

The focus on achieving independence from family care leads to the
problem of finding alternative sheltered residential care for disabled
people, who desire and need close confiding relationships to assist in
daily support and stress management. Most community-based
programmes, such as the Wisconsin model, depend on an extensive
provision of supervised residential accommodation for persons with
disability associated with mental disorders. However, the focus is on
individualised living arrangements, rather than grouping disabled
persons into potentially high-stress units. Although attempts to
secure the support of landlords and friendly neighbours produces
occasional informal carers, case managers are frequently left as the
key confidants and community supports for many people living in
non-family settings. Such support is satisfactory when provided
through highly coordinated teams on a 24-hour basis, but very few
community-based services provide such extensive teamwork, and
there is no research to suggest that these alternatives to family care
are any more effective than the natural resources they seek to
replace.

Staff training in community-based settings

In contrast to the unidisciplinary approach favoured by hospital-based approaches, community-based services tend to conduct training of their staff within a multidisciplinary team framework. This training tends to be informal, on-the-job apprenticeship with new team members co-working alongside their experienced colleagues, who demonstrate their skills for the trainees. This produces a team of professionals with a set of core assessment and intervention skills to supplement the specialised skills they have acquired through earlier professional training. Clinical supervision is carried out across disciplines so that nurses may receive supervision from psychologists, psychiatrists from social workers, etc.

While this approach clearly enhances collaboration between team members, and ensures that all staff acquire the practical skills relevant to their everyday practice, the lack of theoretical training and of clear assessment of competence may have limitations, particularly when dealing with difficult cases, where highly refined biopsychosocial management may be necessary to achieve success. Furthermore, there is a tendency for a lack of guiding theory to lead to an excessive dependence on humanistic support, where professionals adopt roles of surrogate family carers and find it difficult to set boundaries between their professional and personal involvement with disabled cases. There is good research evidence to suggest that many disabled people engender intrusive caring responses in their relatives (Hirsch & Leff, 1975; Miklowitz et al, 1983), and it is probable that such over-involved relationships are readily replicated by caring professionals, who are not adequately prepared to handle such situations.

The need for a clear definition of the main skills that characterise the community-based approach, and a curriculum for training staff in the competent deployment of these skills would seem crucial to successful widespread replication of such methods.

Integrated mental health services

The approach that has been developed in Buckingham has been called *integrated care*. A brief overview is provided here that aims to compare and contrast it with the two preceding approaches. The integrated mental health service is an extension of the community-

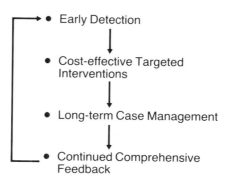

Figure 2.5. A model for integrated care.

based approach that considers the index patient and his or her informal carers as the major contributors to stable recovery from all forms of impairment, disability and handicap associated with mental disorders. This approach seeks to integrate all the efforts of professional and non-professional resources in the community within the vulnerability–stress model for care. The aim is to enhance the efficiency of stress management of the vulnerable person and his or her immediate support network to enable them to achieve full and productive lives in the community with minimal risk of major episodes of mental disorders. In addition to the assertive finding of established cases employed in the community-based approach the integrated service attempts to detect those people most prone to episodes of mental disorders, mainly those with current or past disorders as well as those with early signs of major impairment. Intensive intervention is provided using biopsychosocial methods which, according to the best available research evidence, have been proven to be the most effective. In addition, long-term rehabilitation is provided until all impairment, disability and handicap has been resolved. This cycle of continuing care is illustrated in Figure 2.5.

Where the existing framework of family and primary care is deemed competent, professional intervention aims to maintain and extend these efforts, rather than attempt to replace such resources. One approach to achieving this end involves locating highly-trained mental health specialists within the existing framework of primary health care. The Buckingham Project has been developed as an integrated service that aims to manage all forms of mental disorders in this manner. The aim of the service has been to provide optimal mental health management for all adults between the ages of 16 and 65 years living in a population of around 35,000, and registered with 18 general practitioners in the North Aylesbury Vale. The emphasis has been placed on highly efficient individualised problem-oriented assessment, inclusion of caregivers in all treatment plans, state-of-the-art interventions and continuous long-term assessment aimed at preservation of the quality of life of all members of the community afflicted by the effects of mental disorders.

Four multidisciplinary teams, composed of personnel similar to those allocated to staff a hospital ward, have been integrated within the four functional primary care teams in the area (Figure 2.6). They share premises with the primary care service, and take clinical responsibility for sharing the care of all persons suffering from mental disorders who are registered with each family practice.

In most respects the service is delivered in a manner similar to the community-based approach, with crisis intervention and long-term rehabilitation provided in the natural habitat, making full use of community resources, and facilitating access by those who are disabled to all existing work, social and recreation facilities the community provides for its citizens. The professional services provide direct services for day care or residential care only where current community resources are unable to assist, even when they have been provided with the full support of the mental health team. In practice this reduces the need for specialised institutional resources such as inpatient and day hospital care.

The major differences between this integrated approach and the community-based approach are the extensive education, training and consultative support for patients, informal carers, family practitioners, primary care nurses and other agencies in the community. Within the constraints of their abilities, each person is trained to participate as full members of the team in a manner that is consistent with the vulnerability–stress model. Early detection and intervention of episodes before crises result is considered crucial, and optimal combinations of cost-effective biomedical and psychosocial interventions are employed throughout. Priority is given to people most disabled by mental disorders, but this includes those individuals with persisting anxiety and mood disorders, who are often accorded little attention by services concerned mainly with minimising hospital admissions. Many such individuals have received minimal assistance from hospital-based services despite suffering

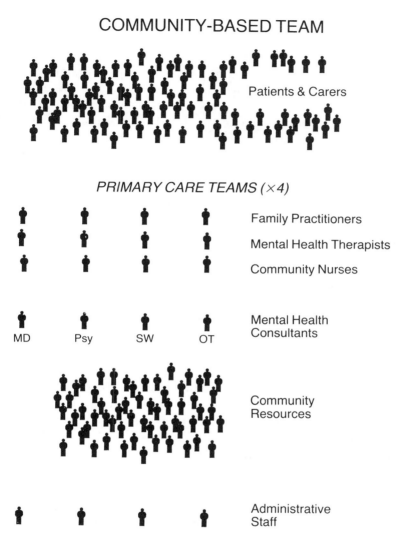

COMMUNITY-BASED TEAM

Patients & Carers

PRIMARY CARE TEAMS (×4)

Family Practitioners

Mental Health Therapists

Community Nurses

Mental Health
Consultants

MD   Psy   SW   OT

Community
Resources

Administrative
Staff

Figure 2.6. A community-based mental health service integrated with primary health care.

disability as severe as any found in the more dramatic presentations of mental disorders.

A further distinction is the emphasis on training mental health professionals in the competent application of a range of assessment and intervention strategies that have been demonstrated as the most effective currently available for most of the common disorders found in the community. A combination of skills-based workshops and supervised practice is provided for all staff on a continuing basis, with assessment of the competence of therapist skills conducted at frequent intervals. Therapists are trained to employ straightforward assessments of levels of impairment, disability and handicap to research standards, so that the benefits that accrue from their therapeutic endeavours can be monitored. All training is conducted across all disciplines to ensure that core skills are maintained, and that a high degree of consistency is achieved throughout the service. As new strategies improve the benefit/cost ratio of those currently employed, further training is provided to ensure that all cases are provided with optimal clinical management.

The following chapters will describe the key aspects of the integrated approach in detail.

Conclusion

The hospital-based approach to community mental health care has several advantages. For example, a centralised location may foster communication between professional staff, and facilitate management. However, there are disadvantages related to accessibility for people who do not reside in the immediate neighbourhood in which the service is sited, a bias towards crisis-management, and an inadequate emphasis on long-term prevention of impairment, disability and handicap. Recent moves to decentralise specific components of the service highlight new problems such as a lack of interdisciplinary collaboration.

The community-based approach offers a longitudinal perspective to community mental health care. The specific needs of people are met in a flexible manner in their own habitats. However, family-style care is not promoted, and non-specific support combined with social casework is the major form of psychosocial intervention. The approach seems most beneficial in the long-term management of the severely disabled. Excellent research studies clearly demonstrate the benefits and costs of this approach compared with traditional hospital care.

The integrated care model is an extension of the community-based approach that seeks to integrate the contributions of professional and non-professional resources in the community within the vulnerability-stress model of mental disorders. The emphasis is on individualised care, targeted use of biomedical and psychosocial interventions of proven efficacy, and continuous long-term assessment and therapy aimed at stable and lasting recovery including restoration of expected lifestyles of all sufferers of mental disorders and their informal carers. A major component of the approach is extensive education, training and consultation for sufferers, carers, primary care teams and all other agencies and people in the community that are involved in the provision of mental health care.

References

Ambelas A. (1987) Life events and mania: a special relationship? *British Journal of Psychiatry*, **150**, 235–240.
Austin, N.K., Liberman, R.P., King, L.W. & DeRisi, W.J. (1976) A comparative evaluation of two day hospitals. Goal attainment scaling of behaviour therapy vs milieu therapy. *Journal of Nervous and Mental Diseases*, **163**, 253–262.
Bennett, D.H. (1982) What direction for psychiatric day centres? In *The Mind Yearbook 1981/82*, MIND: London.
Brown G.W. & Birley J.L.T. (1968) Crises and life changes and the onset of schizophrenia. *Journal of Health and Social Behaviour*, **9**, 203–214.
Brown G.W. & Harris T.O. (1978) *Social origins of depression: a study of psychiatric disorder in women.* Tavistock, London
Corney, R.H.(1981) Social work effectiveness in the management of depressed women: a clinical trial. *Psychological Medicine*, **11**, 417–423.
Creed F., Black D. & Anthony P. (1989) Day hospital and community treatment for acute psychiatric illness. *British Journal of Psychiatry*, **154**, 300–310.
Dick, D. (1982) Alternatives for the care of the mentally ill in Surrey. Keynote address to Surrey Health Authority Seminar, Brighton.
Falloon I.R.H. & Talbot R.E. (1982) Achieving the goals of day treatment. *Journal of Nervous and Mental Disease*, **170**, 279–285.
Falloon I.R.H., Watt D.C. & Shepherd M. (1978) A comparative controlled trial of pimozide and fluphenazine decanoate in the continuation therapy of schizophrenia. *Psychological Medicine*, **7**, 59–70.
Fenton F.R., Tessier L., Struening E.L., Smith F.A. & Benoit C. (1981) *Home and hospital psychiatric treatment.* Croom Helm, London.
Ghosh, A., Marks, I.M. & Carr, A.C. (1984). Self-exposure for phobias: A controlled study. *Journal of the Royal Society of Medicine*, **77**, 483–487.
Grad J. & Sainsbury P. (1963) Mental illness and the family. *Lancet*, **i**, 544–547.

58 *Integrated mental health care*

Gudeman J.E. & Shore M. (1984) Beyond deinstitutionalisation. *New England Journal of Medicine*, **311**, 832–836.
Harris, A. 1957. Day hospitals and night hospitals in psychiatry. *Lancet*, **ii**, 729–730.
Hirsch S.R. & Leff J.P. (1975) *Abnormalities in the parents of schizophrenics*. Oxford University Press, Oxford.
Hoult J. (1986) Community care for the acutely mentally ill. *British Journal of Psychiatry*, **149**, 137–144.
Lamb H.R. (1979) The new asylums in the community. *Archives of General Psychiatry*, **36**, 129–134.
Lamb H.R. & Goerzel V. (1971) Discharged mental patients: Are they really in the community? *Archives of General Psychiatry*, **24**, 29–34.
Leff J.P. & Vaughn C.E. (1985) *Expressed emotion in families*. Guilford Press, New York.
Lewis S.W. & Murray R.M. (1987) Obstetric complications, neurodevelopmental deviance, and schizophrenia. *Journal of Psychiatric Research*, **21**, 413–421.
Liberman R.P., McCann M.J. & Wallace C.J. (1975) Generalization of behaviour therapy with psychotics. *British Journal of Psychiatry*, **129**, 490–496.
Linn, M.W., Caffey, E.M., Klett, J., Hogarty, G.E. & Lamb, H.R. (1979) Day treatment and psychotrophic drugs in the aftercare of schizophrenic patients: A Veterans Administrative cooperative study. *Archives of General Psychiatry*, **36**, 1955–1066.
Marks I.M. (1985) Controlled trial of psychiatric nurse therapy in primary care. *British Medical Journal*, **290**, 1181–1184
May P.R.A. (1968) *Treatment of schizophrenia*. Science House, New York.
McGill, C.W., Falloon, I.R.H., Boyd, J.L., & Wood-Siverio, C. (1983) Family education interventions in the treatment of schizophrenia. *Hospital and Community Psychiatry*, **34**, 934–938.
Miklowitz D., Goldstein M.J. & Falloon I.R.H. (1983) Premorbid and symptomatic characteristics of schizophrenics from families with high and low levels of expressed emotion. *Journal of Abnormal Psychology*, **92**, 359–367.
Miklowitz D.J., Goldstein M.J., Nuechterlein K.H., Snyder K.S. & Mintz J. (1988) Family factors and the course of bipolar affective disorder. *Archives of General Psychiatry*, **45**, 225–231.
Mitchell, A.R.K. (1983) Psychiatrists and GPs: Working together. *Psychiatry in Practice*, **10**, 15–19.
Mosher L.R. & Burti L. (1989) *Community mental health: principles and practice*. Norton, New York.
Mosher L.R. & Menn A.Z. (1978) Community residential treatment for schizophrenia: Two-year follow-up. *Hospital & Community Psychiatry*, **29**, 715–723.
Pasamanick B., Scarpitti F. & Dinitz S. (1967) *Schizophrenics in the community: An experimental study in the prevention of hospitalization*. Appleton-Century-Crofts, New York.

Paykel E.S., Mangen S.P., Griffith J.H. & Burns T.P. (1982) Community psychiatric nursing for neurotic patients: A controlled trial. *British Journal of Psychiatry*, **140**, 573–581.

Polak P.R. & Kirby M.W. (1976) A model to replace mental hospitals. *Journal of Nervous and Mental Disease*, **162**, 13–22

Robson M.H., France R. & Bland M. (1984) Clinical psychologist in primary care: controlled clinical and economic evaluation. *British Medical Journal*, **288**, 1805–1807.

Shepherd, M., Cooper, B., Brown, A.C. & Kalton, G.W. (1966). *Psychiatric illness in general practice*. Oxford University Press, London.

Stein L.I. & Diamond R.J. (1985) The chronic mentally ill and the criminal justice system: When to call the police. *Hospital & Community Psychiatry*, **36**, 271–274.

Stein L.I. & Test M.A. (1980) Alternative to mental hospital treatment: I. Conceptual model, treatment program, clinical evaluation. *Archives of General Psychiatry*, **37**, 392–397.

Stein L.I. & Test M.A. (eds.) (1985) *Training in the community living model – A decade of experience*. Plenum Press, New York.

Strathdee G. & Williams P. (1984) A survey of psychiatrists in primary care. *Journal of the Royal College of General Practitioners*, **34**, 615–618.

Tarrier N., Vaughn C.E., Lader M.H. & Leff J.P. (1979) Bodily reactions to people and events in schizophrenia. *Archives of General Psychiatry*, **36**, 311–315.

Tennant C. & Andrews G. (1978) The pathogenic quality of life event stress in neurotic impairment. *Archives of General Psychiatry*, **35**, 859–863.

Test M.A. & Stein L.I. (1980) Alternative to mental hospital treatment. II. Social cost. *Archives of General Psychiatry*, **37**, 409–412.

Vaughn C.E. & Leff J.P. (1976) The influence of family and social factors on the course of psychiatric illness. A comparison of schizophrenic and depressed neurotic patients. *British Journal of Psychiatry*, **129**, 125–137.

Warner R. (1985) *Recovery from schizophrenia*. Routledge & Kegan Paul, Boston, pp 287–289.

Weisbrod B., Test M.A. & Stein L.I. (1980) An alternative to mental hospital treatment: III. Economic cost-benefit analysis. *Archives of General Psychiatry*, **37**, 400–405.

Williams, P. & Balestrieri, M. (1989) Psychiatric clinics in general practice: Do they reduce admissions? *British Journal of Psychiatry*, **154**, 67–71)

Wykes T. & Wing J.K. (1982) A ward in a house: Accommodation for 'new' long-stay patients. *Acta Psychiatrica Scandinavica*, **56**, 315–330.

3
Effective therapeutic strategies

Overview

In this chapter we review in greater detail a major issue concerning service development. This involves the choice of effective therapeutic strategies to meet efficiently the current needs of the community.

The development of an integrated mental health service should be guided throughout by two clear principles:

1. That every person suffering from a mental disorder as defined by one of the major international classification systems,* who is registered as a patient of a family medical practitioner in the local community is able to receive the most effective clinical management of his or her disorder, until such time as that person moves from the area and/or changes to a family practice outside the designated community. Where family practice is not well established, catchment populations may be defined by other criteria, such as street addresses. However, such criteria tend to be much less satisfactory and tend to impair the accessibility of treatment resources to people in boundary areas.

2. That the effectiveness of the major therapeutic strategies employed by the service would be measured for each case to provide validation for the choice. This assessment would be not merely based upon their efficacy in reducing symptom impairment, but also in resolving psychological and social disability and handicaps. The

---

* The *Diagnostic and Statistical Manual* of the American Psychiatric Association, Third Edition, revised in 1985, DSM-IIIR, or *The International Classification of Diseases* of the World Health Organisation, 10th Edition, ICD–10, are the two latest major classification systems employed throughout the world.

initial choice of the major strategies would be guided by evidence of scientific validation of their efficacy in replicated controlled outcome studies with groups of patients suffering from similar patterns of morbidity. In other words, the clinical management of each patient is considered a field test of the efficacy of a specific therapeutic strategy. Where the choice exists between two or more treatment strategies of equal potency, the following considerations would affect the choice:

i Efficiency of the two approaches – the most efficient in terms of therapist time, training and community costs, including consumer acceptability, would be chosen.
ii Unwanted effects – the strategy with evidence for the least risk of unwanted effects is chosen, including restrictions placed upon the lifestyles of the individual or his/her carers.
iii Additional benefits – the approach that showed evidence of most benefits to the patient, caregiver or community, other than those associated directly with the targeted therapeutic goal, is chosen.

Therapeutic strategies that lack scientific validation of their effectiveness have no place in current mental health service practice. Nor, indeed, do strategies that, although effective, have been superseded by more potent or more efficient methods. Decisions about the deployment of therapeutic resources must be made purely on the basis of scientific data supporting their benefits and costs, and must remain free of ideological or philosophical constraints, apart from those associated with ethical considerations. Discrimination should be purely along scientific lines and devoid of any consideration of age, sex, intelligence, social class, race, language or any other factor, unless specific controlled, replicated treatment research studies conclusively indicate such discrimination contributes to a consistently superior outcome for a specific sociodemographic subgroup.

While it is clear that adherence to such principles is a task that requires considerable integrity and moral courage, we believe that it is unethical practice not to make every reasonable attempt to do so. In publicly funded health services, such as those national health services in Europe, Scandinavia, Australasia, Canada, and the Veterans' Administration in the United States, consumers should have a right to expect that the public funds that they provide through taxation are deployed with maximum efficiency to resolve their specific needs. The needs of the health care agencies that serve as the

Table 3.1. *Prevalence of major mental disorders*

Major affective disorders	5.7%
Anxiety disorders	9.8%
Schizophrenic disorders	1.0%

Note: Derived from the six-month prevalence data of the NIMH epidemiological catchment area study of 9543 people in three US cities (Myers et al, 1984).

providers of that service, both physical and emotional, are not insignificant, but should always be considered as secondary to those of the consumer. Thus, the service should be led by the realistic demands of the consumer, not by the self-interest of the provider.

To set such a high standard makes one an easy prey to human fallibility, and throughout this book the highly critical reader will be aware of case examples that may deviate slightly from these principles. We frequently excuse ourselves on the grounds of inadequate research to guide us, or mismanagement by the systems that support us, or other failings. However, at no time should we be prepared to accept these excuses, without planning contingencies for resolving these issues. Thus, at times we must take a clear advocacy role on behalf of our consumers by seeking development of more effective therapeutic strategies, improved research studies, or more efficient management systems.

Selection of major therapeutic strategies

Epidemiological studies of DSM-III diagnostic categories (or their equivalents) reveal that the three main categories of mental disorders in communities are anxiety disorders, affective disorders and schizophrenic disorders (Table 3.1). Substance misuse and personality disorders are regarded as secondary disorders in the DSM-III classification, and appear as major vulnerability factors that complicate the clinical management of the primary mental disorders. Another category of disorders that is not included in the recent epidemiological surveys are the adjustment disorders. These DSM-III, Axis 1 disorders include a range of abnormal anxiety and depressive states that appear to be precipitated by major stresses, and are not sufficiently severe to meet the criteria for major affective or anxiety disorders. Recent studies have suggested that these conditions may contribute to major clinical and social morbidity and often follow chronic recurring or persistent courses (Dobler-Mikola & Angst, 1989; Kiloh et al, 1988). People with these adjustment disorders are not commonly admitted to inpatient units but are a major source of outpatient and family practice consultations. For these reasons we have included them in this discussion.

It is evident that an effective mental health service to a community should be judged primarily on the efficacy of its clinical management of these major mental disorders. In order to establish the current status of treatment methods for these conditions we will conduct a brief, selective review of the controlled outcome studies of the specific strategies that have demonstrated their effectiveness in the clinical management of each of these conditions.*

Adjustment disorders

These are disorders which are defined in terms of abnormal, usually excessive, mood and behavioural responses to stressful life events. The classification of these disorders is relatively new. They were previously included primarily within classifications of anxiety and depressive disorders. As a result there has not as yet been time to complete a body of controlled outcome studies that clearly demonstrates effective treatment strategies of these disorders using the current classification. These disorders comprise the main body of mental disorders seen by family practitioners, who consider them mild forms of anxiety and depression. However, the clear association between the onset of the disorder and major environmental stresses leads them to provide brief supportive counselling, all too frequently accompanied by tranquillising drugs to assist with problems of sleep

---

* Readers interested in more detailed discussions, that include assessments of the quality of the research methods used in these studies are urged to read the detailed reports of the Australian Department of Health Quality Assurance Project commisioned by the Australian Department of Health, and directed by Professor Gavin Andrews under the aegis of the Royal Australian and New Zealand College of Psychiatrists, published in *The Australian and New Zealand Journal of Psychiatry*, 1982–85.

disturbance or excessive tension (Catalan & Gath, 1985; Coleman & Patrick, 1978; Locke et al, 1967; Shepherd et al, 1966).

In common with many mental health professionals and the lay public, a disorder that is clearly stress-related, or occurs in the context of a physical illness, is often dismissed by primary care physicians and social workers as less significant than one where the provoking factors are less overt, or 'endogenous' (Andrews et al, 1977; Corney, 1981; Freeling et al, 1985). Because most of these disorders tend to remit once the stressful situation has been resolved, few are referred to busy outpatient services with waiting lists longer than two or three weeks. However, a proportion of cases progress to more severe episodes, and where stressors persist the course may be unremitting (Brugha et al, 1990; Goering et al, 1983).

The persistence or recurrence of environmental stressors that appear to provoke vulnerability to these disorders may be associated with relatively straightforward factors, such as inadequate housing and social deprivation (Clare, 1982). However, the manner in which individuals adjust to environmental stress through their repertoire of coping behaviour may play a major role in determining the mental health outcomes associated with adverse life circumstances (Brugha et al, 1990). Thus, people who are considered to have personality disorders that result in relatively ineffective coping strategies, and those who resort to misuse of alcohol, drugs and food as a primary means of coping with life stress, may be among those most vulnerable to continuing impairment, disability and handicap that results from adjustment disorders.

Some studies of psychological interventions have undoubtedly included many cases that would be now classified as adjustment disorders. Perhaps the most relevant of these was the Temple University comparative study of behaviour therapy and psychotherapy (Sloane et al, 1975). This study compared behaviour therapy and psychoanalytic psychotherapy with a four-month waiting list control in a mixed group of psychiatric outpatients suffering from a range of neurotic, adjustment and personality disorders. Although neither active treatment produced significantly more benefits than the reduction in symptoms accomplished merely by waiting in the expectation of receiving treatment, the results favoured the behavioural approach, particularly in terms of relief of the target presenting symptoms. However, on the basis of current research, it must be concluded that there is no specific therapeutic strategy available for this group of conditions, that is more effective than the benefits of natural community support systems.

Nevertheless, a major concern is the proportion of such cases that progress to major affective, anxiety, somatoform or schizophrenic disorders. The task of discriminating between those likely to run a benign remitting course and those likely to escalate is exceptionally difficult, and certainly one that is unlikely to be clearly understood by the average family practitioner, particularly within the time constraints of such consultations. Thus, in addition to devising efficient means of ensuring rapid recovery from the impairment of adjustment disorders, it is important to examine methods of screening for those persons most vulnerable to escalation and to recognise states that may be the prodromal phases of more severe disorders (Fava et al, 1988, 1990; Fava & Kellner, 1991; Herz & Melville, 1980; Murphy et al, 1989). These procedures will be described in detail in Chapter 4.

However, it may be important to recognise the value of assessing these conditions and monitoring their progress. Evidence that stress may play an aetiological role in most forms of mental disorder, particularly in depressive disorders where persons have predisposing vulnerability (Brown & Harris, 1978), would suggest that brief screening with follow-up may have a preventative impact, by detecting prodromal features of depression at an early stage so that effective interventions can be started at an early phase of the disorder (Falloon et al, 1989). But, it must be stressed that such a procedure is not yet validated, and therefore, despite the apparent commonsense formulation, substantial resources should not be diverted from their deployment in areas where efficacy is clear.

Adjustment to stressful life circumstances is seldom isolated to an individual in a community. Most major life events place demands on a wider social network, particularly family units. Events such as bereavements, marital break-up, serious illness, and job loss all impinge directly on all household members. Despite research that indicates that intimate social support appears a key predictor of morbidity, most interventions have employed psychodynamic psychotherapy approaches that focus exclusively on the coping mechanisms and vulnerability factors of the individuals who present for treatment, with very limited reference to their families and friends. Strategies that also address the stresses of the natural social support systems may prove more effective.

Much more controlled outcome research is urgently needed in this area, where unvalidated and poorly regulated counselling approaches are burgeoning. Bereavement counselling, post-divorce counselling, counselling of the victims of assault and of disasters and generic stress management are among the many ventures that have sprung up in recent years (Balestrieri et al, 1988). It is likely that this work does have some effect in preventing mental disorders. One controlled study of women who had experienced a recent bereavement suggested that counselling by a psychiatrist lowered morbidity, particularly in people who had poor social supports (Raphael, 1977). Many studies of disaster victims have suggested that similar counselling may reduce the development of post-traumatic stress disorders (Turner, 1991). Brief problem solving with family pracitioners proved effective in dealing with adjustment disorders presenting with tension and anxiety symptoms (Catalan & Gath, 1985). It is possible that relatively straightforward approaches such as those employed in that study may prove as beneficial as more complex psychotherapies for most cases. However, until replicated controlled studies provide validation for these methods, and, furthermore, they have demonstrated benefit/cost ratios that support their feasibility in clinical settings, such methods should be encouraged only when they are provided by voluntary community workers and agencies, not as part of the mainstream mental health service (Lamb & Zusman, 1981). Of course such efforts may derive considerable benefit from skilled mental health professionals, who may *volunteer* their personal expertise in the training of counsellors, as well as assist with the research and development of these methods.

Anxiety disorders

Anxiety symptoms are endemic in all communities. Mental disorders associated with such symptoms are considered to be present when the responses to a feared object or situation are excessive, and either lead to continuing distress or social disability. These disorders cover a wide range of conditions and severity including phobic disorders, panic disorders, generalised anxiety (GAD) and obsessive compulsive disorders (OCD). Somatoform disorders, where irrational anxiety about physical health is a prominent feature, may also be included in this discussion. This diversity means that several therapeutic strategies may be necessary for their management.

A large body of research has demonstrated reduction in clinical features of anxiety in phobic disorders, including agoraphobia, when a variety of desensitisation techniques have been applied (Agras, 1985; Emmelkamp, 1982; Marks, 1987; Quality Assurance Project, 1982). The most efficient strategy appears to be real-life exposure to the feared object or situation (Marks, 1976; 1987). This involves coaching the patient to remain in contact with the specific stimulus that provokes anxiety until they experience a reduction in the anxiety response. The way in which the person is exposed to the feared stimulus may be varied according to that person's needs, some preferring a rapid and more stressful approach, others a more gradual approach over a longer period. Recent studies suggest that these methods can be successful in many instances where the patient carries out the specific strategies in the absence of the therapist, either alone, or with the assistance of a family member or friend (Mathews et al, 1981; Ghosh et al, 1987; Falloon et al, 1977). However, much of this research has not yet been replicated.

Drug therapy, particularly with tricyclics, appears to add to the benefits of exposure strategies where anxiety is associated with panic attacks (Zitrin et al, 1983; Agras, 1985). However, in common with the problems associated with long-term benzodiazepine therapy and the less frequently prescribed monoamine-oxidase inhibitors (MAOIs), recurrences of anxiety symptoms frequently occur when these drugs are withdrawn (Tyrer, 1988; Kelly, 1970; Sheehan et al, 1984). The relative benefits of the therapeutic strategies that have been most frequently investigated in controlled trials of agoraphobia are summarised in Figure 3.1.

Panic attacks and intense anxiety that do not appear to be associated with specific environmental triggers, have until recently been treated most effectively by drugs (Klein et al, 1978). Controlled studies have shown equal efficacy for benzodiazepine derivatives, beta blockers and tricyclics (Klerman, 1986). However, these drugs merely control anxiety, have a wide range of unpleasant side effects, and are difficult to withdraw (Rickels et al, 1980).

Although earlier attempts to develop alternative non-drug strategies were not as potent as drugs, at least in the short term (see Figure 3.2), some recent series of studies have indicated that psychological approaches to anxiety management that involve combinations of

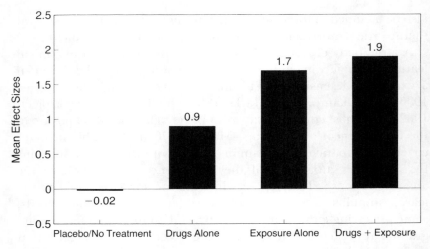

Figure 3.1. Benefits of therapeutic strategies for agoraphobia. (From Mattick et al, 1990.)

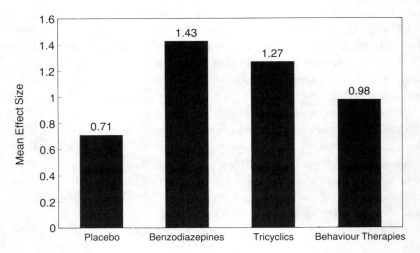

Fig. 3.2. Benefits of therapeutic strategies for generalised anxiety and panic. (From Quality Assurance Project, 1985 a.)

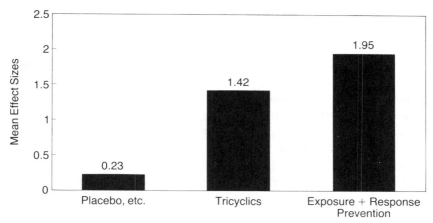

Figure 3.3. Benefits of therapeutic strategies for obsessive-compulsive disorders. (From Quality Assurance Project, 1985b.)

muscular relaxation, respiratory control, and cognitive strategies may be as effective as drug therapies without the risk of unwanted effects (Ost, 1987; Butler et al, 1987; Clark, 1986; Mattick et al, 1990). However, drugs remain an alternative strategy for persons with anxiety that remains disabling, despite effective application of psychological treatments. Fortunately, there is no evidence to suggest that drugs reduce the efficacy of psychological strategies, although there is little evidence that the combination produces any additional benefits (Marks, 1983; Zitrin et al, 1983).

Social skills training, which combines role-played rehearsal and real-life practice of interpersonal interaction (a form of exposure), is an effective therapeutic strategy for persons with social phobias (Butler et al, 1984). Drugs appear to have little benefit for these disorders (Falloon et al, 1981). However, social anxiety is extremely complex and relatively few controlled studies of treatment strategies have been conducted.

Obsessive compulsive disorder, OCD, is one of the most disabling mental disorders (Black, 1974). Although its prevalence in the community is similar to that of schizophrenia, and it tends to follow a more persistent course, it has been neglected in the planning of most hospital-based services. Figure 3.3 shows that the outlook has improved somewhat in recent years. The most helpful strategy appears to combine exposure to the triggers of obsessional responses with self-controlled prevention of those responses, such as repeated hand-washing or counting rituals (Beech & Vaughan, 1978; Foa & Goldstein, 1978; Marks, 1987; Rachman & Hodgson, 1986). However, obsessional thought disturbance has proved much more refractory to treatment of all kinds (Foa, 1979; Quality Assurance Project, 1985b). Cognitive strategies, such as thought stopping, where the person is trained to develop means of stopping a repeated thought, and the contrasting strategy of satiation, where the person attempts to maximise the unwanted thought until it disappears, appear to have short-term benefits but have not been consistently effective in controlled studies (Kirk, 1983). Controlled studies of the efficacy of tricyclic drugs in OCD have produced similarly inconsistent results. Marks (1983) has argued that the main benefits of tricyclic drug therapy for cases of OCD is derived from their ability to relieve associated depressive features, and that their effects on the specific obsessional symptoms is minimal. However, to date there have been very few studies that have compared drug treatments with cognitive behavioural strategies. Thus, we have concluded that each case of OCD should be viewed as a single case experiment with combinations of psychological and drug strategies applied in attempts to reduce morbidity according to clearly formulated hypotheses (see Turner & Beidel, 1988).

The somatoform disorders are relatively common in the community, contributing substantially to disability, as well as consuming substantial general health resources. These consist of persons with irrational fears about their health, as well as those who manifest their emotional distress in predominantly physiological responses, such as gastrointestinal, respiratory and neuromuscular dysfunction and pain. There is a dearth of evidence of effective strategies for these disorders (Quality Assurance Project 1985c). However, there is a consensus that traditional general medicine is of limited benefit, and that the reassurance usually provided may indeed exacerbate the disorder (Warwick & Salkovskis, 1985).

Longitudinal studies show that the gains achieved after relatively brief therapy for anxiety disorders tend to be maintained for at least two years (O'Sullivan & Marks, 1991). However, full remission of anxiety symptoms, as well as associated disability and handicaps is seldom reported, and is probably much less common than the research literature would suggest (Barlow, 1984). Treatment benefits are least readily obtained in the complex anxiety disorders such as agoraphobia, social phobia, and in obsessive compulsive disorder.

Exacerbations of anxiety disorders appear associated with environmental stress factors, both discrete life events (Tennant & Andrews, 1978), and family stress (Hafner, 1986). To date, methods to prevent such exacerbations have not been researched. It would seem that the repeated application of treatment strategies in booster sessions at the time of minor exacerbations may sustain progress (O'Sullivan & Marks, 1991). However, it is probable that stress management, possibly including carers may prove effective. This may be achieved more readily where family members or other key carers are engaged in education about the disorders and the application of psychological strategies in the initial phases of therapy (Mathews et al, 1981; Falloon et al, 1977).

Despite their high prevalence, relatively few attempts have been made to prevent the onset of anxiety disorders, or to intervene at an early stage. This latter strategy may be expected to have benefits in preventing the development of extensive lifestyle adjustments that are often made to adapt to anxiety symptoms. Such coping mechanisms themselves often contribute to the handicaps associated with the disorders, and may delay recovery (Wolpe, 1977). It is probable that early intervention may prevent at least some of the severe disability associated with the major disorders.

Recent studies have revealed an incidence of suicide in anxiety disorders similar to that associated with affective disorders (Allgulander & Lavori, 1991). Delay in recognising this association is undoubtedly due to the frequent co-morbidity of anxiety and depressive disorders. However, the despair associated with severe anxiety states should not be underestimated, and effective, comprehensive treatment sought without delay. Although there is good evidence that many cases remit without specific treatment (Rachman & Wilson, 1980), that phenomenon is evident in most mental (and physical) disorders, and should not provide support for lengthy waiting lists.

Affective disorders

These disorders include episodes of persistent mood disturbance where inappropriate expressions of unhappiness or elation predominate. This mood change is usually accompanied by activity level changes with sleep and appetite disturbances and physical symptoms. Variation in the course and severity of episodes is frequent,

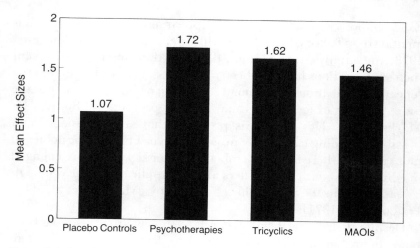

Figure 3.4. Benefits of therapeutic strategies for 'endogenous' depression. (From Quality Assurance Project, 1983.)

with mild depression one of the most common psychiatric symptoms in community surveys (Shepherd et al, 1966; Andrews et al, 1977). The association between physical symptoms and depressive episodes makes diagnosis difficult for family practitioners, resulting in substantial delays in treatment of many cases (Kupfer et al, 1989). The association between depressive states and various endocrine abnormalities, such as Cushing's syndrome and hypothyroidism, anaemias and viral disorders, as well many drug side effects, necessitates adequate medical assessment of all suspected cases. However, there is a tendency for milder episodes to remit within a few weeks without specific treatment. Efforts to delineate different syndromes of depression have been made mainly on the basis of whether the episode appears to be triggered directly by a major life event, or tends to arise without obvious psychosocial precipitants. Unfortunately, such issues are seldom clear cut. Furthermore, efforts to distinguish between patterns of symptoms, are similarly difficult to apply in practice. These issues make the assessment of the effectiveness of treatment approaches very difficult, particularly as most research studies have included cases of widely different symptom patterns and severity levels. It can be seen from Figures 3.4 and 3.5 that a substantial difference in the choice of treatment strategies is associated with the different syndrome patterns.

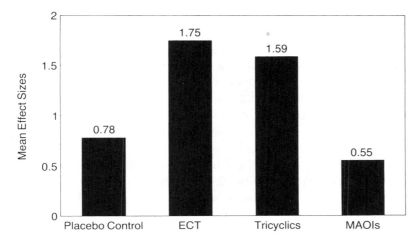

Figure 3.5. Benefits of therapeutic strategies for 'neurotic' depression. (From Quality Assurance Project, 1983.)

Tricyclic drugs and their derivatives have been the mainstay of antidepressant therapy. Their effectiveness is limited by a slow action and poor tolerance of effective doses by many persons (Kessler 1978). Alternative drugs have proved less toxic, but controlled studies have shown little overall benefits from newer and more expensive preparations (Wager & Klein, 1988). Monitoring of plasma levels of antidepressant drugs has not yet contributed to any major improvements in efficacy (Rowan et al, 1984). In general, no clear relationships between therapeutic effects and the blood levels of the drugs or their active metabolites have been found, and the presence of side effects is an effective clinical guideline for dosage adjustment.

Psychological interventions have demonstrated similar effectiveness to drug therapy in mild to moderate depression (see Figure 3.5), particularly where psychosocial factors are most clearly associated with pathogenesis (Teasdale, 1988). Three main strategies have been studied: activity scheduling, cognitive restructuring and interpersonal skills training. Despite considerable interest in the cognitive approaches there is no evidence that this is generally the most potent strategy. A recent large collaborative study has revealed similar short-term potency for these approaches, as well as for tricyclics (Elkin et al, 1989). However, tricyclics and the non-behavioural interpersonal psychotherapy proved more effective than cognitive therapy with more severe episodes. Several studies suggest additional benefits from the combination of tricyclics and psychological interventions (Elkin et al, 1989; Blackburn et al, 1981). At the moment outcome tends to be measured in terms of changes on the combined scores of depression rating scales, despite hypotheses that the various drug and psychosocial strategies have selective effects on specific symptoms. Efforts to conduct studies that aim to tease out the relative benefits of the various treatments for the differing syndromes of depression are in their infancy, but may be expected to produce useful guidelines for clinical practice (Quality Assurance Project, 1983; Shotsky et al, 1991).

At the moment is seems reasonable to conclude that the most effective clinical management of depressive episodes involves a targeted approach that endeavours to provide specific intervention strategies for specific symptoms – hormones and general medical intervention for specific medical problems; tricyclics for sleep, appetite, agitation and retardation; cognitive restructuring for unrealistic and worrying thoughts; activity scheduling for lack of constructive or pleasing activity; and interpersonal skills training for enhancing pleasurable social interaction. This problem-specific approach can be employed in the intensive treatment of more severe forms of depression, and appears remarkably similar to that generally advocated for the hospital management of such episodes, where nursing procedures, occupational therapy, psychology programmes are employed in combination with drug therapy.

Studies of the clinical management of persisting depressive disorders, such as dysthymia, have yet to demonstrate any specific benefits from drug or psychosocial interventions, although it has been suggested that treatment failure is most often due to a lack of persistence with the intervention strategies (Wager & Klein, 1988). The erroneous belief that almost all depressive states remit spontaneously after relatively brief episodes have undoubtedly contributed to intervention studies that tend to be extremely brief, and seldom examine outcome in terms of recovery from the episodes.

Electroconvulsive therapy (ECT) has been shown to be more effective than placebo (anaesthetic without convulsions) in severe episodes when there is failure to respond to the drugs and psychological combination (Janicak et al, 1985; Kendell, 1981). As Figure 3.5 suggests ECT appears most effective in episodes of 'endogenous' depression, where negative thoughts reach delusional intensity

(Northwick Park, 1984; Paykel, 1979). Despite its detractors, serious side effects are relatively rare and reversible. However, whereas the benefits of ECT are achieved more rapidly than through drug therapies, these advantages appear to be lost at follow-up (Medical Research Council, 1965). Little is known about the mechanisms for the effectiveness of ECT, and consequently, whether the same effects could be induced by less invasive drug and psychosocial interventions (Crow, 1979). Further studies are needed to elucidate more clearly the comparative benefits of ECT, drug and psychosocial treatments in the treatment of the different symptom patterns of depressive disorders.

Despite evidence that depressive disorders have a high rate of recurrence (Keller et al, 1982; Kiloh et al, 1988), remarkably few studies have examined methods for preventing recurrent episodes. Tricyclics have been effective in reducing the rate of recurrence in cases where residual symptoms persist, but the benefits of long-term drug prophylaxis are poorly understood (Prien et al, 1984). Cognitive behavioural interventions have been associated with lowered recurrence rates (Teasdale, 1988; Miller et al, 1989). However, the association between environmental stress and depressive episodes that has been well documented in studies of life events (Brown & Harris, 1978; Ambelas, 1987) and family tension (Vaughn & Leff, 1976; Hooley et al, 1986) has not yet led to the development of stress management strategies that may prevent episodes. Three studies have shown the benefits of family-based management of depressive episodes, but further study of strategies that aim to enhance the stress management capacity of persons vulnerable to depressive disorders are needed before these approaches can be considered consistently effective (O'Leary & Beach, 1990; Glick et al, 1985; Jacobson, 1988).

It should be remembered that patients are not the only persons who suffer as a result of a depressive episode, family members and close friends often share the burden, and may succumb to mental disorders themselves (Fadden et al, 1987). Although there is not yet research evidence to support its efficacy, the provision of education about the nature of depression and its clinical management to patients and carers is generally considered a crucial aspect of treatment. This may assist in the early detection of exacerbations and the efficient application of intensive treatment to prevent serious recurrences (Kupfer et al, 1989).

A major problem in the clinical management of depressive disorders is the increased risk of suicide. Suicidal thoughts are common in depression, but fortunately relatively few persons translate this negativistic thinking into self-destructive behaviour. Self-destructive actions are frequently associated with major stress in persons who lack effective problem solving skills to cope with overwhelming personal crises (Hawton & Catalan, 1987). In some cases this stress-related behaviour is associated with depressive episodes and adjustment disorders. The complex relationships between suicidal thinking and decisive action make assessment of the risk of death or serious injury exceptionally difficult. Consequently the management of such a state is often confused. There is a tendency to employ protective measures that aim to prevent the person attempting to harm himself, rather than to explore the cognitive and emotional factors that may provide a more specific predictor of the risk of suicidal actions (Beck et al, 1979). Hopelessness, helplessness and frustration associated with ineffective attempts to solve the perceived problems of the distressed person may be relieved by repeated problem solving that assists the sufferer to consider alternative strategies to those involving self-destructive acts (Hawton & Kirk, 1988). Of course where the depressive syndrome is clearly present, other biological and psychosocial strategies will be targeted to major symptoms. However, it has been noted that many severely depressed persons commit suicide when they appear to be recovering from the major physical symptoms. No entirely satisfactory explanations for this observation have been proposed, but it is possible that the negativistic thinking is somewhat independent of biological factors, and may require independent psychological treatment.

Persisting dysphoric mood states, classified as dysthymic disorders in DSM-III, are major problems in the community. The lack of effective drug treatment causes many people to seek alternative help from that afforded by psychiatric services and they remain frequent attenders at primary care facilities. It has been hypothesised that persons suffering these states have difficulty coping with stress and are often prone to increase, rather than decrease, their ambient stress levels as a consequence of their inadequate attempts to cope. The major life events that they experience are often dependent on their own behavioural responses to pre-existing stress. For example, a woman who perceives her husband's lack of attention to her needs as a stress may leave him, taking her young children with her, and subsequently find herself unable to cope with single parenthood, inadequate finances and housing, all far greater stresses than the original interpersonal problem, which may have been relieved by marital counselling. Assisting such persons to improve their coping capabilities through problem solving and interpersonal skills training appears to be effective (Falloon et al, 1977), but further controlled research must be completed before such an approach can be recommended on a widespread basis.

Manic episodes are considered among the most difficult disorders to manage. Their onset is often acute, sometimes associated with major stresses, and frequently results in patterns of behaviour that are embarrassing for family, friends, and, when recovered, the sufferers themselves. Tranquillising drugs may dampen down the most extreme features of hyperactivity and excitability, but the effects are relatively slow. Lithium may have additional tranquillising benefits in the acute phase. The lack of a rapid, dramatic response often leads to administration of excessive doses of drugs with toxic effects that exacerbate the condition. The highly pleasureable experiences usually associated with the disorder make many patients reluctant to collaborate with treatment that aims to reduce euphoria, and not infrequently leads to a depressed mood, particularly in bipolar cases.

In the absence of dramatically effective pharmacological measures, psychosocial strategies that assist the manic person to achieve some measure of self-control are vital. Although hospital nursing practice often achieves considerable calming of persons experiencing manic episodes, very few such strategies have been studied systematically, and at the moment there is no evidence for the efficacy of any specific psychosocial interventions.

Lithium salts have demonstrated their benefits in reducing the risk of recurrent episodes of mania. However, these benefits are limited to a 50% reduction in the risk of recurrence, and further limited by long-term toxic effects (Prien & Gelenberg, 1989). The use of serial monitoring of serum levels maximises the benefit/cost ratio through maintaining dose levels within a narrow therapeutic window (Schou, 1989).

The association between stress factors and manic episodes is less well established than with depression (Sclare & Creed, 1990; Miklowitz et al, 1988), and consequently there are no published studies of the benefits of stress management approaches. One controlled study is currently in progress following evidence that the addition of behavioural family therapy to lithium prophylaxis resulted in a reduced risk of recurrent episodes (D.J. Miklowitz, personal communication).

The clinical management of bipolar disorders, where manic and depressive episodes alternate, has been improved by the prophylactic effects of lithium therapy, which tends to diminish the severity of recurrent mood swings. To all intents and purposes the management of episodes is similar to that of unipolar conditions. Early detection of episodes with intervention prior to the onset of the most disturbing presentations of symptoms when collaboration between patients, carers and professionals is most difficult, may enable episodes to be somewhat blunted. It is probable the the regular assessment associated with monitoring lithium levels may contribute in this way. However, to date no studies of early intervention have been conducted.

Schizophrenic disorders

These disorders are characterised by the presence of cognitive deficits, including hallucinations, delusions and thought interference. They have a wide range of severity with courses that range from brief episodes with minimal disability, relapses and remissions, to persisting states that resemble profound dementias with severe social dysfunction (Shepherd et al, 1989).

Over the past 30 years the clinical management of these disorders has improved dramatically. This has occurred in three phases: first, the provision of psychosocial rehabilitation resources has enabled even those persons most handicapped by the disorder to lead a constructive life in the community; second, the discovery of the tranquillising effects of the neuroleptic drugs has enabled most acute episodes of schizophrenia to be modified significantly; thirdly, the development of stress management, often involving persons caring for the patient, has reduced the risk of recurrent episodes when combined with long-term drug prophylaxis (Strachan, 1986; Falloon & Shanahan, 1990).

Neuroleptic drug therapy and a calm supportive environment are the basis for facilitating recovery from florid psychotic episodes (Quality Assurance Project, 1984). Three out of four cases derive

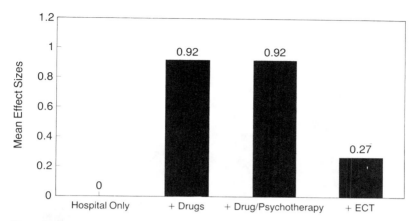

Figure 3.6. Benefits of therapeutic strategies for acute schizophrenic episodes. (From Quality Assurance Project, 1984.)

substantial benefits from this regimen (Goldberg et al, 1965), although full remission of symptoms occurs in less than two-thirds (Shepherd et al, 1989), with a further third suffering persistent cognitive disturbance and associated deficits of mood, motivation and behavioural responses (sometimes termed 'negative' symptoms). Figure 3.6 shows that no additional benefits have been demonstrated when traditional psychotherapies have been added to optimal drug treatment, ECT has a very limited role, and there is little evidence that a typical hospital milieu contributes to the effectiveness of specific drug treatment. Of course it is crucial that treatment is adequately supervised in a safe, and supportive environment. Alternatives to hospital environments have now been demonstrated as feasible locations for effective intensive care (Mosher & Burti, 1989; see Chapter 4).

There is no evidence for any differential benefits for any particular drug, and the choice of drug is based upon the side effects profile experienced by each person (Schooler & Severe, 1984). Neurological side effects resembling Parkinson's disorder may be helped by antiparkinsonism drugs, but these drugs have their own unpleasant effects in turn, and because most of the unwanted effects can be reduced by adjusting the dose of the neuroleptic, long-term administration is seldom recommended (Davis et al, 1980). More serious effects, such as tardive dyskinesia, are less readily treated, and have led to substantial efforts to develop drugs that can be administered

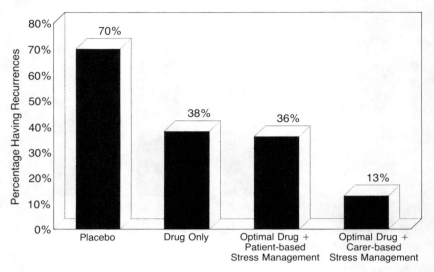

Figure 3.7. Benefits of therapeutic strategies for preventing recurrent episodes. (From Falloon & Shanahan, 1990.)

safely for several years without major risks (Marder & Van Putten, 1988). Until such drugs have been established it seems crucial that drug therapy is carefully targeted to each person's changing needs, so that benefits are maximised and unwanted effects minimised. A major advance in establishing optimal drug dosage has resulted from the measurement of plasma levels (Van Putten et al, 1991). Therapeutic windows have been established for the most commonly used drugs that ensure that benefits are maximised, and unwanted effects associated with excessive doses avoided.

The continuation of drug therapy once florid episodes have improved has reduced the rate of recurrence in the first year after an episode from around 70% of all cases to 30–40% (Falloon & Shanahan, 1990; Figure 3.7). The risk of a major exacerbation is further reduced where psychosocial stress management is added to optimal drug therapy to between 10 and 20% of all cases. The most effective approaches have combined education about the nature of schizophrenia and its treatment with psychological methods that aim to enhance the efficiency of problem solving of not merely the person suffering the disorder, but his or her immediate caregivers, so that all forms of environmental stress may be dealt with effectively (Liberman & Mueser, 1988; Strachan, 1986).

The combined benefits of drug prophylaxis and stress management do not persist after the treatment is withdrawn, necessitating continued application (Falloon & Shanahan, 1990). The provision of psychological treatment as well as drug therapy can be tapered off to a 'low dosage' regimen after the first 3–6 months of care, but boosters of greater intensity may be needed to counter periods of major life stress (Brown & Birley, 1968; Birley & Brown, 1970), or other times when symptom exacerbation may emerge (Herz et al, 1991). Patients and their caregivers, including family practitioners, may be trained to recognise the early signs of impending exacerbations so that delays in providing effective crisis management may be minimal (Birchwood et al, 1989; Herz & Melville, 1980; Carpenter & Heinrichs, 1983). There is some evidence that such an approach may facilitate clinical and social recovery when it is sustained for at least two years (Falloon, 1985). Low dosage prophylaxis has tended to prove more feasible than intermittent drug strategies, where withdrawal may itself occasionally contribute to psychotic exacerbations (Simpson et al, 1976; Jolley & Hirsch, 1989; Herz et al, 1991).

Although clinical remission and social recovery are closely associated, the aim of treatment should always be primarily to restore function. Psychosocial rehabilitation extends the benefits achieved by symptomatic treatment so that disability and handicap is minimised (Hall, 1989; Liberman, 1988). A wide range of strategies have been effectively employed to assist persons who have suffered schizophrenia to return to a normal lifestyle, even when the impairments of the disorder persist. There is adequate research to support the benefits of social skills training (Wallace & Liberman, 1985; Hogarty et al, 1986), life skills training (Paul & Lentz, 1977), family-based behavioural and cognitive strategies (Falloon, 1985) and long-term social casework (Hogarty et al, 1974; 1979) in improving social functioning and sustaining life in the community. Controlled case reports suggest that specific psychological interventions can be tailored for patients with persisting hallucinations and delusions, that assist the patients to cope with those problems (Tarrier, 1991). However, there are insufficient studies of groups of cases to provide firm evidence of the efficacy of these approaches.

The provision of adequate social supports, such as housing, day care, sheltered employment and vocational training has received little evaluative scrutiny (Creed et al, 1989; Falloon et al, 1987). Uncontrolled reports suggest that such methods are highly benefic- ial, but further studies are needed to confirm the cost-effectiveness of these projects and to determine the relative benefits of the wide variety of methods advocated so that persons responsible for meeting the needs of disabled persons in the community can be met in the most efficient manner.

There is accumulating evidence that the prognosis for schizophre- nia may be improved when effective treatment is started early in the course of the disorder (Wyatt, 1991). However, diagnosis at an early stage may be extremely difficult, particularly in cases where the onset is gradual. Early detection is further hampered by the stigma that is still attached to this disorder in most communities and the notion that this remains an incurable disorder. There is considerable need for updating the diagnostic skills of the professional community and improved public awareness of the benefits of modern treatment. Improved detection and early intervention with optimal combi- nations of biomedical and psychosocial treatment strategies offers hope of improved recovery rates, and reductions in long-term disability and handicap (Lewis & Murray, 1987; Falloon, 1992).

Conclusion

This brief review of the state-of-the-art management of the major forms of mental disorders indicates that highly effective treatment strategies are currently available for most conditions. Controlled research studies have replicated the specific benefits of the major intervention approaches used to treat acute episodes of anxiety, affective and schizophrenic disorders. These have included drug therapies, psychological strategies and effective combinations of the these approaches.

With the exception of lithium salts in the stabilising of mood swings, drugs do not appear to have highly specific anxiolytic, antidepressant or antipsychotic properties, and are best utilised to ameliorate targeted symptoms, rather than heterogeneous syn- dromes. Within each of the three major groups of drugs there is little evidence for differential effectiveness. Thus, the choice of drug should be based upon the side effect profile for individuals, and secondarily on the cost, particularly where long-term administration is proposed.

Psychological treatment strategies are similarly generic in their application. Specific strategies are targeted for specific problems and tailored according to individual needs. Controlled research has been conducted mainly on behavioural and cognitive methods, and relatively few studies have examined the differential benefits of different strategies as well as the comparative costs. Costs of psychological interventions should include the cost of training therapists, which in the case of some complex cognitive and psychoanalytic approaches can be extensive. When compared with drug therapies, the more labour intensive psychological approaches may appear more costly in the short term, but may have benefits that continue long after the intensive therapeutic input has been completed, whereas most drug therapies require continuous administration to sustain their beneficial action. For these reasons it is dangerous to draw any conclusions about relative costs and benefits, unless careful economic studies have been completed. At the present moment few cost-benefit studies have been conducted so that the main criterion for selecting treatment strategies should be the effectiveness of each strategy in resolving the specific problem to which it is being targeted.

Major replications, particularly those involving multi-site collaboration, have demonstrated that therapists can be trained to administer the main approaches in a consistently effective manner. However, even when relatively straightforward drug therapies are applied in clinical practice, there is considerable variation in their application. Such deviation is more likely with psychosocial strategies of greater complexity, and is likely to reduce the effectiveness of the approaches. Thus, training therapists to those levels of competence where specific benefits of therapeutic approaches are known to be achieved in a consistent fashion must be a major priority for any mental health service to a community. Limited research has been conducted to compare various training approaches, or to establish measures of therapist competence that can be employed to ensure that effective application of treatment strategies is maintained. However, it is clear that few mental health professionals are equipped with the full range of treatment strategies that we have

reviewed here, and few services can take pride in providing the
people with mental disorders that they serve with the most effective
clinical management strategies. The integrated approach to mental
health care ensures that every person experiencing a major mental
disorder receives the optimal combination of those biomedical and
psychosocial strategies that have demonstrated their efficacy in
controlled clinical trials.

References

Agras W.S. (1985) *Panic, facing fears, phobias and anxiety.* W.H. Freeman,
    San Francisco.
Allgulander C. & Lavori P.W. (1991) Excess mortality among 3302
    patients with 'pure' anxiety neurosis. *Archives of General Psychiatry,*
    48, 599–602.
Ambelas A. (1987) Psychologically stressful events in the precipitation of
    manic episodes. *British Journal of Psychiatry,* **135**, 15–21.
Andrews G., Schonell M. & Tennant C. (1977) The relation between
    physical, psychological and social morbidity in a suburban
    community. *American Journal of Epidemiology,* **105**, 324–329.
Balestrieri, M., Williams P. & Wilkinson G. (1988) Specialist mental
    health treatment in general practice: a meta-analysis. *Psychological
    Medicine,* **18**, 711–717.
Barlow D. (1984) The psychosocial treatment of anxiety disorders:
    current status and future directions. In J.B. Williams & R.L. Spitzer
    (Eds.) *Psychotherapy Research.* Guilford Press, New York.
Beck A.T., Rush A.J., Shaw B.F. & Emery G. (1979) *Cognitive therapy of
    depression.* Guilford Press, New York.
Beech H.R. & Vaughan M. (1978) *Behavioural treatment of obsessional states.*
    Wiley, New York.
Birchwood M., Smith J., MacMillan F., Hogg B., Prasad R., Harvey C.
    & Bering S.(1989) Predicting relapse in schizophrenia: the
    development and implementation of an early signs monitoring
    system using patients and families as observers, a preliminary
    investigation. *Psychological Medicine,* **19**, 649–656.
Birley J.L.T. & Brown G.W. (1970) Crises and life changes preceding
    the onset or relapse of acute schizophrenia: Clinical aspects. *British
    Journal of Psychiatry,* **116**, 327–333.
Black A. (1974) The natural history of obsessional neurosis. In H.R.
    Beech (Ed.) *Obsessional states.* Methuen, London.
Blackburn I.M., Bishop S., Glen A.I.M., Whalley L.J. & Christie J.E.
    (1981) The efficacy of cognitive therapy in depression: a treatmen†

trial using cognitive therapy and pharmacotherapy, each alone and in combination. *British Journal of Psychiatry*, **139**, 181–189.

Brown G.W. & Birley J.L.T. (1968) Crises and life changes and the onset of schizophrenia. *Journal of Health and Social Behaviour*, **9**, 203–214.

Brown G.W. & Harris T.O. (1978) *The social origins of depression.* Tavistock Press, London.

Brugha T.S., Bebbington P.E., MacCarthy B., Sturt E., Wykes T. & Potter J. (1990) Gender, social support and recovery from depressive disorders: a prospective clinical study. *Psychological Medicine*, **20**, 147–156.

Butler G, Cullington A., Hibbert G., Klimes I. & Gelder M. (1987) Anxiety management for persistent generalised anxiety. British Journal of Psychiatry, **151**, 535–542.

Butler G., Cullington A., Munby M., Amies P. & Gelder M.G. (1984) Exposure and anxiety management in the treatment of social phobia. *Journal of Consulting and Clinical Psychology*, **52**, 642–650.

Carpenter W.T. & Heinrichs D.W. (1983) Early intervention, time-limited, targeted pharmacotherapy of schizophrenia. *Schizophrenia Bulletin*, **9**, 43.

Catalan J. & Gath D.H. (1985) Benzodiazepines in general practice: a time for decision. *British Medical Journal*, **290**, 1374–1376.

Clare A.W. (1982) Social aspects of ill-health in general practice. In A.W. Clare & R.H. Corney (Eds.) *Social work and primary health care*, pp 9–22. Academic Press, London.

Clark D.M. (1986) Cognitive therapy of anxiety. *Behavioural Psychotherapy*, **14**, 283–294.

Coleman J.V. & Patrick D.L. (1978) Psychiatry and general health care. *American Journal of Public Health*, **68**, 451–457.

Corney R.H. (1981) Social work effectiveness in the management of depressed women: a clinical trial. *Psychological Medicine*, **11**, 417–423.

Creed F., Black D. & Anthony P. (1989) Day-hospital and community treatment for acute psychiatric illness: a critical appraisal. *British Journal of Psychiatry*, **154**, 300–310.

Crow T. (1979) The scientific status of electro-convulsive therapy. *Psychological Medicine*, **9**, 401–408.

Davis J.M., Schaffer C.B., Killian G.A. et al. (1980) Important issues in the drug treatment of schizophrenia. *Schizophrenia Bulletin*, **6**, 70–87.

Dobler-Mikola A. & Angst J. (1989) Depressive syndromes in field studies: problems of case definition. *World Psychiatric Association Bulletin*, **1**, 7–12.

Elkin I., Shea, T., Watkins J.T., Imber S.D., Sotsky S.M. Collins J.F., Glass D.R., Pilkonis P.A., Leber W.R., Docherty J.P., Fiester S.J. & Parloff M.B. (1989) National Institute of Mental Health treatment of depression collaborative research program: General effectiveness of treatments. *Archives of General Psychiatry*, **46**, 971–982.

Emmelkamp P.M.G. (1982) *Phobic and obsessive-compulsive disorders.* Plenum Press, New York.

Fadden G., Bebbington P. & Kuipers L. (1987) Caring and its burdens: a study of the spouses of depressed patients. *British Journal of Psychiatry*, **151**, 660–667.

Falloon I.R.H. (1985) *Family management of schizophrenia*. Johns Hopkins University Press, Baltimore.

Falloon I.R.H. (1992) Early intervention for first episodes of schizophrenia. *Psychiatry*, **55**, 4–15.

Falloon I.R.H., Lindley P., McDonald R. & Marks I.M. (1977) Social skills training of outpatient groups: a controlled study of rehearsal and homework. *British Journal of Psychiatry*, **131**, 599–609.

Falloon, I.R.H., Lloyd, G.G. & Harpin, R.E. (1981) The treatment of social phobia: real-life rehearsal and non-professional therapists. *Journal of Nervous and Mental Disease*, **169**, 180–184.

Falloon I.R.H. & Shanahan W.J. (1990) Community management of schizophrenia. *British Journal of Hospital Medicine*, **43**, 62–67.

Falloon I.R.H., Shanahan W., Krekorian H.A.W. & Laporta M. (1989) Prevention of major depressive episodes: early intervention with family stress management. Paper presented at the annual meeting of the Social, Community and Rehabilitation Section of the Royal College of Psychiatrists, London, February 1989.

Falloon I.R.H., Wilkinson G., Burgess J. & McLees S. (1987) Evaluation in psychiatry: Planning, developing and evaluating community-based mental health services for adults. In D. Milne (Ed.), *Evaluating mental health practice*. Croom Helm, London.

Fava G.A., Grandi S., Canestrari, R. (1988) Prodromal symptoms in panic disorder with agoraphobia. *American Journal of Psychiatry*, **145**, 1564–1567.

Fava G.A., Grandi S., Canestrari R. & Molnar G. (1990) Prodromal symptoms in primary major depressive disorder. *Journal of Affective Disorders*, **19**, 149–152.

Fava G.A. & Kellner R. (1991) Prodromal symptoms in affective disorders. *Americal Journal of Psychiatry*, **148**, 823–830.

Foa E.B. (1979) Failures in treating obsessive-compulsives. *Behaviour, Research & Therapy*, **17**, 821–829.

Foa E.B. & Goldstein A. (1978) Continuous exposure and complete response prevention in obsessive-compulsive neurosis. *Behavior Therapy*, **9**, 821–829.

Freeling P., Rao B.M., Paykel E.S., Sireling L.I. & Burton R.H. (1985) Unrecognised depression in general practice. *British Medical Journal*, **290**, 1880–1883.

Ghosh A., Marks I.M. & Carr A.C. (1987) Therapist contact and outcome of self-exposure for phobias: a controlled study. *British Journal of Psychiatry*, **152**, 234–238.

Glick I.D., Clarkin J.F., Spencer J.H., Haas G.L., Lewis A.B., Peyser J., De Mane N., Good-Ellis M., Harris E. & Lestelle V. (1985) A controlled evaluation of Inpatient Family Intervention: I.

Preliminary results of the six-month follow-up. *Archives of General Psychiatry*, **42**, 882–886.

Goering P., Wasylenski D., Lamce W. & Freeman S.J. (1983) Social support and post-hospital outcome for depressed women. *Canadian Journal of Psychiatry*, **28**, 612–623.

Goldberg S.C., Klerman G.L., Cole J.O. (1965) Changes in schizophrenic psychopathology and ward behavior as a function of phenothiazine treatment. *British Journal of Psychiatry*, **111**, 120–133.

Hafner, R.J. (1986) *Marriage and mental illness*. Guilford Press, New York.

Hall J. (1989) Chronic psychiatric handicaps. In K. Hawton et al. (Eds.) *Cognitive behaviour therapy for psychiatric problems*, pp 313–333. Oxford University Press, Oxford.

Hawton K. & Catalan J. (1987) *Attempted suicide; a practical guide to its nature and management*. Oxford University Press, Oxford.

Hawton K. & Kirk J. (1988) Problem solving. In K. Hawton, P.M. Salkovskis, J. Kirk & D.M. Clark (Eds.) *Cognitive behaviour therapy for psychiatric problems*, Oxford University Press, Oxford.

Herz M.I., Glazer W.M., Mostert M.A., Sheard M.A., Szymanski H.V., Hafez H., Mirza M. & Vana J. (1991) Intermittent vs maintenance medication in schizophrenia: two-year results. *Archives of General Psychiatry*, **48**, 333–339.

Herz M.I. & Melville C. (1980) Relapse in schizophrenia. *American Journal of Psychiatry*, **137**, 801–805.

Hogarty G.E., Anderson C.M., Reiss D.J., Kornblith S.J., Greenwald D.P., Javna C.D. & Madonia M.J. (1986) Family psycho-education, social skills training and maintenance chemotherapy in the aftercare treatment of schizophrenia. I. One-year effects of a controlled study on relapse and expressed emotion. *Archives of General Psychiatry*, **43**, 633–642.

Hogarty, G.E., Goldberg, S.C., Schooler, N.R. & Ulrich, R.F. (1974). Drug and sociotherapy in the aftercare of schizophrenic patients. II. Two-year relapse rates. *Archives of General Psychiatry*, **31**, 603–608.

Hogarty G.E., Schooler N.R., Ulrich R.F. et al. (1979) Fluphenazine and social therapy in the aftercare of schizophrenic patients: relapse analysis of a two-year controlled trial. *Archives of General Psychiatry*, **36**, 1283–1294.

Hooley J.M., Orley J. & Teasdale J.D. (1986) Levels of expressed emotion and relapse in depressed patients. *British Journal of Psychiatry*, **148**, 642–647.

Jacobson N.S. (1988) Cognitive-behavioural marital therapy for depression. Paper presented at World Congress of Behaviour Therapy, Edinburgh, September 1988.

Janicak P.G., Davis J.M., Gibbons R.D., Ericksen S., Chang G. & Gallagher D. (1985) Efficacy of E.C.T. – a meta-analysis. *American Journal of Psychiatry*, **142**, 297–302.

Jolley A.G. & Hirsch S.R. (1989) Brief intermittent neuroleptic prophylaxis for stable schizophrenic outpatients. *Schizophrenia Research*, **2**, 508.

Keller M.B., Shapiro R.W.., Lavori P.W. & Wolfe N. (1982) Relapse in major depressive disorder: analysis with the life table. *Archives of General Psychiatry*, **39**, 911–915.

Kelly D., Guirguis W. Frommer E. et al. (1970) Treatment of phobic states with antidepressants: A retrospective study of 246 patients. *British Journal of Psychiatry*, **116**, 387–398.

Kendell R.E. (1981) The present status of electroconvulsive therapy. *British Journal of Psychiatry*, **139**, 265–283.

Kessler K.A. (1978) Tricyclic antidepressants: mode of action and clinical use. In M.A. Lipton, A. DiMascio & K.F. Killam (Eds.) *Psychopharmacology: A generation of progress*. Raven Press, New York.

Kiloh L.G., Andrews G. & Neilson M. (1988) The long-term outcome of depressive illness. *British Journal of Psychiatry*, **153**, 752–757.

Kirk, J.W. (1983) Behavioural treatment of obsessive-compulsive patients in routine clinical practice. *Behaviour Research and Therapy*, **21**, 57–62.

Klein D.F., Zitrin C.M. & Woerner M. (1978) Anti-depressants, anxiety, panic and phobia. In M. Lipton, A. DiMascio & K.F. Killam (Eds.) *Psychochpharmacology: A generation of progress*, Raven Press, New York.

Klerman G.L. (1986) Current trends in clinical research on panic attacks, agoraphobia and related anxiety disorders. *Journal of Clinical Psychiatry*, **47**, 37–39.

Kupfer D.J., Frank E. & Perel J.M. (1989) The advantage of early treatment in recurrent depression. *Archives of General Psychiatry*, **46**, 771–775.

Lamb H.R. & Zusman J. (1981) A new look at primary prevention. *Hospital and Community Psychiatry*, **32**, 843–848.

Lewis S.W. & Murray R.M. (1987) Obstetric complications, neurodevelopmental deviance, and schizophrenia. *Journal of Psychiatric Research*, **21**, 413–421.

Liberman R.P. (1988) *Psychiatric rehabilitation of chronic mental disorders*. American Psychiatric Press, Washington, D.C.

Liberman R.P. & Mueser K.T. (1988) Psychosocial treatment of schizophrenia. In S. Kaplan & B.J. Sadock (Eds.) *Comprehensive textbook of psychiatry*, 5th ed. Williams & Wilkins, Baltimore.

Locke B.Z. Finucane D.L. & Hassler I. (1967) Emotionally disturbed patients under care of private nonpsychiatric physicians. *American Psychiatric Association: Psychiatric Research Report*, **22**, 235–248.

Marder, S.R. & Van Putten, T. (1988) Who should receive clozapine? *Archives of General Psychiatry*, **45**, 865–867

Marks I.M. (1976) The current state of behavioral psychotherapy: Theory and practice. *American Journal of Psychiatry*, **133**, 253–261.

Marks, I.M. (1983) Are there anticompulsive and antiphobic drugs? Review of the evidence. *British Journal of Psychiatry*, **143**, 338–347.

Marks, I.M. (1987) *Fears, phobias and rituals.* Oxford University Press, Oxford.

Mathews A.M., Gelder M.G. & Johnson D.W. (1981) *Agoraphobia: Nature and treatment.* Guilford Press, New York.

Mattick R.P., Andrews G., Hadzi-Pavlovic D. & Christensen H. (1990) Treatment of panic and agoraphobia: An integrative review. *Journal of Nervous and Mental Disease,* **178**, 567–576.

Medical Research Council (1965) Clinical trial of the treatment of depressive illness. *British Medical Journal,* **i**, 881–886.

Miklowitz D.J., Goldstein M.J., Nuechterlein K.H., Snyder K.S. & Mintz J. (1988) Family factors and the course of bipolar affective disorder. *Archives of General Psychiatry,* **45**, 225–231.

Miller I.W., Norman W.H. & Keitner G.I. (1989) Cognitive-behavioral treatment of depressed patients: Six- and twelve-month follow-up. *American Journal of Psychiatry,* **146**, 1274–1279.

Mosher L.R. & Burti L. (1989) *Community mental health: principles and practice.* Norton, New York.

Myers J.K., Weissman M.M., Tischler G.L., Holzer C.E., Leaf P.J., Orvaschel H., Anthony J.C., Boyd J.H., Burke J.D., Kramer M. & Stoltzman R. (1984) Six-month prevalence of psychiatric disorders in three communities; 1980 to 1982. *Archives of General Psychiatry,* **41**, 959–967.

Murphy J.M., Sobol A.M., Olivier D.C., Monson R.R., Leighton A.H. & Pratt L.A. (1989) Prodromes of depression and anxiety: The Stirling County study. *British Journal of Psychiatry,* **155**, 490–495.

Northwick Park ECT Trial (1984) Predictors of response to real and simulated ECT. *British Journal of Psychiatry,* **144**, 227–237.

O'Leary K.D. & Beach S.R.H. (1990) Marital therapy: A viable treatment for depression and marital discord. *Americal Journal of Psychiatry,* **147**, 183–186.

Ost L.G. (1987) Applied relaxation: description of a coping technique and review of controlled studies. *Behaviour Research and Therapy,* **25**, 397–410.

O'Sullivan G. & Marks I. (1991) Long-term follow-up of agoraphobia, panic and obsessive-compulsive disorders. In R. Noyes (Ed.) *Handbook of anxiety,* Vol. 4. Elsevier, Amsterdam.

Paykel E.S. (1979) Predictors of treatment response. In E.S. Paykel and A. Coppen (Eds.) *Psychopharmacology of Affective Disorders.* Oxford University Press, Oxford.

Paul G.C. & Lentz R.J. (1977) *Psychosocial treatment of chronic mental patients.* Harvard University Press, Cambridge, MA.

Prien R.F. & Gelenberg A.J. (1989) Alternatives to lithium for preventive treatment of bipolar disorder. *American Journal of Psychiatry,* **146**, 840–848.

Prien R.F., Kupfer D.J., Mansky P.A., Small J.G., Tuason V.B., Voss C.B. & Johnson W.E. (1984) Report of the NIMH Collaborative Study Group comparing lithium carbonate, imipramine, and a lithium combination. *Archives of General Psychiatry,* **41**, 1096–1104.

Quality Assurance Project. (1982) A treatment outline for
    agoraphobia. *Australian and New Zealand Journal of Psychiatry*, **16**, 25–33.
Quality Assurance Project. (1983) A treatment outline for depressive
    disorders. *Australian and New Zealand Journal of Psychiatry*, **17**, 129–
    146.
Quality Assurance Project. (1984) Treatment outlines for the
    management of schizophrenia. *Australia and New Zealand Journal of
    Psychiatry*, **18**, 19–38.
Quality Assurance Project. (1985a) Treatment outlines for the
    management of anxiety states. *Australia and New Zealand Journal of
    Psychiatry*, **19**, 138–151.
Quality Assurance Project. (1985b) Treatment outlines for the
    management of obsessive-compulsive disorders. *Australia and New
    Zealand Journal of Psychiatry*, **19**, 240–253.
Quality Assurance Project. (1985c) Treatment outlines for the
    management of somatoform disorders. *Australia and New Zealand
    Journal of Psychiatry*, **19**, 397–407.
Rachman S.J. & Hodgson R.J. (1986) *Obsessions and compulsions*. Prentice
    Hall, Englewood Cliffs, N.J.
Rachman S.J. & Wilson G.T. (1980) *The effects of psychological therapy*.
    Pergamon, Oxford.
Raphael B. (1977) Preventive intervention with the recently bereaved.
    Archives of General Psychiatry, **34**, 1450–1454.
Rickels K., Case C.G. & Diamond L. (1980) Relapse after short-term
    drug therapy in neurotic patients. *International Pharmacopsychiatry*, **15**,
    186–192.
Rowan P.R., Paykel E.S., Marks V., Mould G. & Bhat A. (1984) Serum
    levels and response to amitryptiline in depressed outpatients.
    Neuropsychobiology, **12**, 9–15.
Schooler N.R. & Severe J.B. (1984) Efficacy of drug treatment for
    chronic schizophrenic patients. In M. Mirabi (Ed.) *The chronically
    mentally ill: research and services*. Spectrum, New York.
Schou M. (1989) Lithium prophylaxis: myths and realities. *American
    Journal of Psychiatry*, **146**, 573–576.
Sclare P & Creed F. (1990) Life events and the onset of mania. *British
    Journal of Psychiatry*, **156**, 508–514.
Sheehan D.V., Coleman J.H., Greenblatt D.J. et al. (1984) Some
    biochemicaal correlates of panic attacks with agoraphobia and their
    response to treatment. *Journal of Clinical Psychopharmacology*, **4**, 66–75.
Shepherd, M., Cooper, B., Brown, A.C. & Kalton, G.W. (1966).
    Psychiatric illness in general practice. Oxford University Press, Oxford.
Shepherd M., Watt D., Falloon I., Smeeton N. (1989) The natural
    history of schizophrenia: a five-year follow-up study of outcome and
    prediction in a representative sample of schizophrenics. *Psychological
    Medicine Monograph 16*, Cambridge University Press, Cambridge.
Shotsky S.M., Glass D.R., Shea M.T., Pilkonis P.A., Collins J.F., Elkin
    I., Watkins J.T., Imber S.D., Leber W.R., Moyer J. & Oliveri M.E.

(1991) Patient predictors of response to psychotherapy and pharmacotherapy: Findings in the NIMH treatment of depression collaborative research program. *American Journal of Psychiatry*, **148**, 997–1008.

Simpson G.M., Varga E. & Haher E.J. (1976) Psychotic exacerbations produced by neuroleptics. *Diseases of the Nervous System*, **37**, 367–369.

Sloane R.B., Staples F.R., Cristol A.H., Yorkston N.J. & Whipple K. (1975) *Psychotherapy versus behavior therapy*. Harvard University Press, Cambridge, MA.

Strachan A.M.(1986) Family intervention for the rehabilitation of schizophrenia: towards protection and coping. *Schizophrenia Bulletin*, **12**, 678–698.

Tarrier N. (1991) Behavioural psychotherapy and schizophrenia: the past, present, and the future. *Behavioural Psychotherapy*, **19**, 121–130.

Teasdale J. (1988) Cognitive therapy for depression: the state of the art. Paper presented at the World Congress of Behaviour Therapy, University of Edinburgh, September 1988.

Tennant C. & Andrews G. (1978) The pathogenic quality of life event stress in neurotic impairment. *Archives of General Psychiatry*, **35**, 859–863.

Turner R.M. & Beidel D.C. (1988) *Treating obsessive-compulsive disorder*. Pergamon Press, New York.

Turner S.W. (1991) Post-traumatic stress disorder. *Hospital Update*, August, 644–649.

Tyrer P. (1988) Prescribing psychotropic drugs in general practice. *British Medical Journal*, **296**, 588–589.

Van Putten T., Marder S.R., Wirsching W.C., Aravagiri M. & Chabert N. (1991) Neuroleptic plasma levels. *Schizophrenia Bulletin*, **17**, 197–216.

Vaughn C.E. & Leff J.P. (1976) The influence of family and social factors on the course of psychiatric illness. *British Journal of Psychiatry*, **129**, 125–137.

Wager S.G. & Klein D.F. (1988) Drug therapy strategies for treatment-resistant depression. *Psychopharmacology Bulletin*, **24**, 69–74.

Wallace C.J. & Liberman R.P. (1985) Social skills training for patients with schizophrenia: a controlled clinical trial. *Psychiatry Research*, **15**, 239–247.

Warwick H.M.C. & Salkovskis P.M. (1985) Reassurance. *British Medical Journal*, **290**, 1028.

Wolpe J. (1977) Inadequate behavioral analysis: the Achilles' heel of outcome research in behavior therapy. *Journal of Behavior Therapy and Experimental Psychiatry*, **8**, 1–4.

Wyatt R.J. (1991) Neuroleptics and the natural course of schizophrenia. *Schizophrenia Bulletin*, **17**, 325–351.

Zitrin C.M., Klein D.F., Woerner M.G. & Ross D.C. (1983) Treatment of phobias. I: Comparison of imipramine hydrochloride and placebo. *Archives of General Psychiatry*, **40**, 125–138.

4

Early detection of major mental disorders

Background

Assessing the needs of mental health care in a community begins with the detection of cases of all people experiencing mental disorders in the population served. It is crucial that potential cases gain access to the specific interventions that lead to a reduction in their morbidity in a highly efficient manner. As well as defining those people who have the characteristic impairments, disabilities and handicaps associated with mental disorders, it is important to ensure that this screening process is as accurate as possible, so that all cases are recognised with minimal delay and a minimal number of people who do not have mental disorders are not included in the selection of cases. The latter may have impairment, disability or handicap similar to that associated with mental disorders, but are less likely to benefit from the specific intervention procedures, and indeed may be harmed by their application. Because the criteria for defining mental disorders emphasise cognitive-behavioural abnormalities that cannot yet be supported by specific pathophysiological characteristics (e.g. blood tests, X-rays etc.), professionals conducting assessments must be highly skilled in the application of these criteria, thereby missing few cases and including few non-cases.

Primary prevention of major mental disorders has not yet been achieved. However, in common with most health problems, treatment of mental disorders appears to be most effective when applied early in their course, and delayed intervention may contribute to higher levels of persisting clinical, social and carer morbidity (Crow et al, 1986). Delays also appear to contribute to difficulty engaging people into treatment, and the need for coercive procedures to ensure treatment for people who are severely depressed or deluded.

Several factors may contribute to delays in achieving effective early intervention. These include peoples' fear about the consequences of having a mental disorder leading to avoidance of consultation with medical services, poor screening by family practitioners, inexact diagnostic assessment by mental health professionals, and inefficient treatment of detected cases. In this chapter the methods we have devised to overcome these problems and to foster early detection and effective treatment of episodes of major mental disorders will be outlined.

Screening by family practitioners

In most health services family practitioners provide the major gatekeeping role. Referrals to specialist services are usually made at the request of the family practitioner, with the exception of major accidental trauma, and long-term case management is monitored by the family practitioner service with whom the great majority of patients are registered. Consultations with the family practitioner are readily accessed and may be requested on a 24-hour basis, every day of the week. As a result, a family practitioner service is likely to consult with almost every patient on an annual basis, particularly if there is any evidence of impaired function. Goldberg and Huxley (1980) suggested that over 90% of all people suffering from mental disorders in the UK consulted their doctors during the course of a year. Similar levels of consultations with primary care services have been noted in other countries (Brodaty & Andrews, 1983; Dilling & Weyrerer, 1984). Despite the often very brief nature of these consultations, and the fact that they are often made expressly for treatment of physical disorders, family practitioners are able to detect around 60% of all mental disorders. In other words, most family practitioners provide reasonably good screening for mental disorders, even in the absence of any formal screening procedures. However, it is evident that many cases are missed, and these are not always minor disorders. Several reasons for this have been proposed. First, people consult their family practitioners primarily when suffering from physical discomfort, and doctors perceive their primary role as detecting life-threatening diseases, rather than dealing with social disability. Some people experiencing depressive and anxiety disorders present with physical manifestations that mask abnormal mental states. These often require great skill in determining the primary pathology, and it is apparent that even when detailed assessments are made by specialised medical services, a substantial proportion of mental disorder is initially misdiagnosed and often mistreated. A typical example of this was a 23-year-old man who attended a cardiology clinic for over a year, receiving extensive tests, including a 10-day period in an inpatient unit, because he complained of intermittent chest constriction, dizziness and palpitations. Only after all tests revealed no cardiac pathology was he referred to the mental health service as a case of suspected hypochondriasis. Immediately, he was recognised as experiencing panic attacks associated with hyperventilation, and after specific anxiety management made a satisfactory recovery.

In addition to missing cases that present with physical complaints, a substantial number of people who suffer from chronic physical disability for whom there is no adequate medical treatment are considered to have mental disorders when none exist. These are often sufferers of chronic and persisting pain, or neurological complaints that do not meet criteria for various syndromes. After medical management has failed to relieve their suffering they are frequently told that they have 'nothing wrong' and are 'imagining' their symptoms. The confusion between such people and sufferers of hypochondriacal syndromes (essentially an irrational fear of having a serious physical disorder) is very common among family practitioners and medical specialists alike. Of course anyone suffering distressing chronic physical discomfort or disability is at risk of developing secondary anxiety and depression, and may require substantial psychosocial counselling to maximise their functioning and minimise handicap.

In the large proportion of consultations that do not result in detection of a mental disorder their management is probably best left in the hands of the medical specialists with consultation from mental health services when necessary. An example of this problem was a 45-year-old woman, who was unable to walk unaided owing to intermittent muscle weakness in her legs. Multiple sclerosis had been suspected, but the diagnosis was not confirmed. Her frequent distressed calls for family practitioners after falls in her home gained her a reputation of a 'problem-patient'. On occasions she told doctors that her life was not worth living and that she had considered suicide. As a result she was considered to have a mental disorder and her management handed over to the mental health service. No mental disorder was detected, but she was clearly distressed by her symptoms and the clinical management she had been receiving. A community occupational therapist arranged for her to use a wheel-chair and to have her home equipped to assist her with her disability. A program of constructive activities was arranged, including attendance at a day centre for the physically disabled. Two years later her disorder had progressed and a definite diagnosis of multiple sclerosis was made.

The association between physical and emotional symptoms appears to confuse many physicians and to lead to frequent misunderstanding between mental health and other medical services. *All major mental disorders have physical symptoms and all major medical disorders have emotional symptoms.* We have attempted to develop a problem-based approach to assessment and treatment that is holistic and minimises pejorative labelling of emotional problems as less important than physical manifestations of disorders. Nevertheless, clear accurate diagnosis of major syndromes of mental disorders is crucial to early and effective intervention.

While sorting out the primary diagnosis of people who present with mixtures of clear-cut physical and emotional symptoms is a complex issue, a more common dilemma facing the family practitioner is deciding when a response to a clear life stress is considered a symptom of a mental disorder. Sleep disturbance, appetite loss, muscular tension, agitation, poor concentration, anxious or unhappy mood, and thoughts of suicide are all common responses to serious life stress. They are also all key features of major mental disorders, all of which are precipitated by environmental stress. The ability to accurately predict those cases where the stress response is a prodromal phase of a major mental disorder would enable effective treatment to be initiated early, and possibly lead to a more benign presentation of a potentially disabling disorder.

Because of the central role of the family practitioner in the initial screening process and subsequent referral on for specialist consultation, a key feature of the integrated approach is very close liaison with family practitioners and an emphasis on training them to identify accurately mental disorders and their prodromal features. Details of this integration in the screening of major mental disorders are provided later in this chapter.

Reducing fear and avoidance of consultation about mental disorders

One of the greatest problems in health care delivery is the fear associated with being diagnosed as suffering from a serious illness. This applies to physical disorders as well as mental disorders. The reasons underlying this fear and the associated avoidance of medical assessment when a person suspects they are suffering from a disorder are complex. As a result the simplistic notions that early intervention can be enhanced merely through multi-media programs of health promotion are likely to meet with disappointing results. In the absence of adequate research on this topic, our experience has led us to conclude that a program that endeavours to address fear and avoidance in a case-by-case manner is more likely to prove effective in meeting this need. We have noted that irrational fears (phobias) are not readily changed by cognitive interventions that merely provide insight into the nature of the fear, unless this understanding is accompanied by behaviour change that involves facing the feared situation and recognising that the consequences can be coped with without overwhelming panic. The integrated approach endeavours to enhance understanding about specific mental disorders, facilitate informal consultation in a non-threatening environment, and provide clinical management that aims to minimise the stress associated with assessment and treatment interventions. The following strategies are employed:

Daily accessibility for consultation, including evenings and weekends: Staff were available to conduct routine assessments at any time throughout the week at the convenience of the person requesting the consultation. In most cases, assessments were conducted within weekday office hours, exceptions being people who worked, particularly those who commuted long distances. A shift system eased the burden for staff, who were able to assess most cases without any inconvenience.

Informal style of requests for consultation: Requests for consultation were all routed through each person's family practitioner with minimal formality. Referral letters were abandoned and replaced with a card entitled *The Community Health Record* (see Appendix 1), that enabled the family practitioner to make brief, pertinent remarks concerning the nature of the problem, reason for consultation, and current clinical management. However, one member of the mental health service was present in the practice throughout clinic times, and wherever feasible was invited to discuss the case with the family practitioner prior to completion of the card. This facilitated appropriate referral to the mental health specialists, and ensured that people who had problems that could be more readily managed by other agencies were referred with minimal delays. For example, couples with marital discord not associated with a mental disorder could be referred for marital counselling, people with social difficulties, such as housing or benefits could be referred to the appropriate social services. If any doubt existed the person was seen jointly with the family practitioner, who always retained the right to request further specialised assessment, including a recommendation that a particular specialist member of the team conduct all or part of the assessment, e.g. a psychologist where a memory deficit was suspected; or a psychiatrist where the case was associated with physical health problems.

Brief discussion with the family practitioner, or other 'screening' agents aimed to define:

1 Nature and duration of disturbed behaviour, mood, cognitive functioning, e.g. are the features suggestive of depressive disorder or merely a person distressed by a recent major stress? Is there evidence that suggests the person is experiencing auditory hallucinations or merely acting a bit strangely?
2 Presence of features that suggest a high risk of a mental disorder; for example, first degree relatives who have had a major mental disorder, developmental disorders, long-term tranquilliser use, drug and alcohol abuse, persisting major life stresses.
3 Current management of any physical disorders, e.g. drugs taken, neuro-endocrine problems.
4 Current management of disturbance by the primary care team, or other agencies.
5 Adequacy of community supports, e.g. caring family or friends.
6 Capacity of primary care team to continue management with specialist back-up where necessary.

The family practitioner is often well informed about the social as well as medical history of cases, and with the assistance of the medical records, may be able to reduce substantially the time needed to secure reliable background information. Detailed medical assessment with a range of laboratory tests may be a vital part of the initial assessment. In such cases the family practitioner is usually the best person to supervise such assessments. Indeed, sometimes the family practitioner may be the most appropriate person to manage the entire assessment and treatment. In these cases specialist members of the mental health team may provide continued supervision and consultation wherever needed. Such mutual understanding has been fostered by daily contact between mental health professionals and family practitioners. The on-duty mental health professional endeavours to speak briefly with each family practitioner before and after each clinic session, and to be accessible for longer consultations when necessary.

It may appear that the service focusses exclusively on consultation with family physicians. This is not the case. The family practitioner remains the gatekeeper for the service, screening cases prior to requesting a second opinion, and keeping lifetime records of each person's physical and mental health. However, if a community nurse, social worker, police or other community agent requests a consultation for a suspected mental health problem, this request is made initially to the family practitioner, who may or may not ask for a second opinion from the mental health specialists. Regular contact is maintained with these agencies, as well as with schools, church groups, voluntary groups and other community supports so that consultation can be facilitated and cases detected at the earliest phase possible. Clinical management is shared with these people in a manner similar to that provided for other informal carers and the primary care professionals.

Minimal delay in establishing initial consultation: Once it has been established that a consultation with the mental health service is appropriate the mental health professional on duty makes contact with the person immediately. It is preferable that this initial contact is made in the family practice offices, but at times this is difficult. A family practitioner may have detected the problem during a domiciliary visit, or late at night, and not considered it an urgent matter. Regardless of the circumstances the family practitioner personally introduces the mental health professional who is on duty for the practice team to the patient. The mental health professional consults with the patient, ensures that immediate crisis assessment and management needs are provided, and arranges further assessment and treatment at a time and location preferred by the person and his/ her carers. This initial personal contact seeks to build rapport with the person and his carers, and to educate them about the nature of the assessment and treatment process. This contact may be no more than 2 or 3 minutes, but may be extended to complete the initial assessment if mutually convenient. Although this is best achieved through a face-to-face meeting, for the reasons outlined above, occasionally this may be conducted over the telephone. However, it should be noted that almost all the people who have refused mental health assessment have been those where personal contact was not made at the point the consultation was requested, and some delay ensued.

Assessment conducted in a non-threatening environment: The two locations where most people prefer to undergo their initial mental health assessments are their homes and their family practitioners' offices. Whenever possible people are invited to nominate the setting where they would prefer to meet with a therapist for their assessment; on occasions these have been the workplace, school, coffee shop, a friend's house, solicitor's office or other venue. The main point is that the locus of assessment is one that the person feels most at ease.

Of course the therapists may feel uneasy conducting assessments in unfamiliar surroundings, particularly if the person they are assessing may be potentially dangerous. It is essential that therapists avoid compromising their ability to relate to people through making arrangements that provoke anxiety. At least two therapists attend any interviews with potentially dangerous people, and such interviews may require careful planning. However, the principle of choosing the least threatening environment for the person who is undergoing assessment may reduce the risk of aggressive behaviour in such cases. Many patients who associate a mental health assessment with a removal of their civil rights and unpleasant incarceration in a mental hospital feel reassured when the therapist visits them at home and treats them in a friendly, respectful manner. The presence of household members during interviews with potentially dangerous people may further protect the therapist from the risk of

assaults. Despite conducting a considerable proportion of assessment interviews in community settings, these procedures appear to
have been successful in reducing the risk of aggressive incidents.
Only one minor assault on a mental health staff member has been
reported in the Buckingham Project during 6 years.

Assessment includes key carers: The initial assessment includes an
interview with key people in the social environment. The aims of this
interview are:

1 To obtain validation for important aspects of your assessment and
   initial formulation and to provide further information when
   necessary.
2 To assess the strengths and weaknesses of home-based support in
   assisting with clinical management.
3 To assess the mental health of other household members, and
   their own vulnerability to develop disorders as a result of the stress
   associated with caring for the disturbed person.

Whereas in cases of mild disorders the assessment of key carers
may last no more than 5–10 minutes, where a major disorder is
suspected a comprehensive interview is conducted with all household members, after which detailed goals are formulated for individuals as well as the living group as a whole. It is assumed that any
people caring for others who are suffering potentially chronic health
problems are themselves vulnerable to stress-induced health problems as a result of long-term strain. Where disorders may be in part
genetically linked, the health risks of blood relatives are heightened
further. The assessment and management of people in these caregiving roles is elaborated further in Chapters 5 and 6.

Efficient preliminary assessment

Although a comprehensive assessment of a person experiencing an
episode of a major mental disorder may extend over several days,
preliminary findings are reported back to the family practitioner as
soon as the therapists have completed the initial consultation with
the person and carers. A brief meeting is scheduled with the family
practitioner, or other people in the primary care services who have
requested the second opinion. A brief discussion about initial

impressions is coupled with systematic notes made on the Community Health Record, which is placed in the person's medical record. These notes include relevant current, past, developmental and social history; provisional diagnosis and preliminary management plan, including recommendations for drug and psychosocial intervention strategies, as well as further assessment plans and medical, psychological and social investigations. Any immediate measures that might be necessary, such as prescription of sedative or tranquillising medication, securing the safety of the patient and carers, the provision of intensive nursing management, etc., are discussed and initiated after the family practitioner has consented to the management plans. Thus, within the integrated model of care, the family practitioner remains the primary case manager throughout, and in instances where disagreements about management occur, is the final arbiter.

Where a major mental disorder is suspected, the team psychiatrist is consulted immediately. The psychiatrist may conduct a conjoint assessment with the therapist and/or family practitioner, or review the preliminary assessment. In such cases the therapist will have completed all relevant parts of the Present State Examination (PSE), and will be prepared to discuss the clinical formulation in detail. The psychiatrist will usually wish to check the reliability of key elements of the mental status and history in a face-to-face meeting with the person and carers, and to clarify the therapist's provisional recommendations about clinical management. In situations where psychological, occupational or social assessment may be similarly relevant, the same procedures for additional consultation are employed. Minimal delays are strongly advocated so that interventions can be instigated with maximal efficiency.* Further discussion about each case is provided at a weekly meeting of each practice team, at which all members of the team meet with the specialist consultants and primary care professionals.

It will be evident that the ease of access to mental health professionals and the speed of response have many benefits in achieving effective screening followed by swift initiation of therapeutic interventions for those people experiencing mental disorders. These procedures are summarised in Figure 4.1.

---

* The specialist consulting members of the service remain readily available for emergency consultations through carrying a relatively small personal caseload, and conducting almost all their clinical work conjointly with other team members.

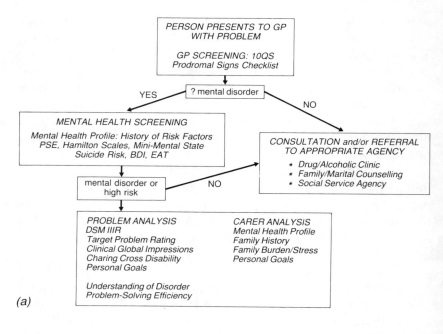

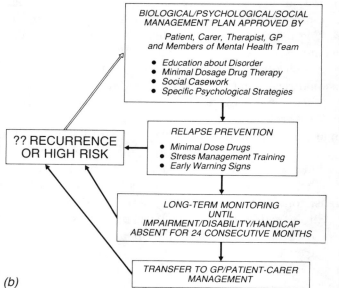

Figure 4.1. (a) *Flowchart of assessment process of an integrated mental health service.* (b) *Flowchart of clinical management process of an integrated mental health service.*

Increasing understanding of specific mental disorders

The role of consumer education is discussed in several chapters throughout this book. It is a core component of the integrated approach. Every person who experiences features of a mental disorder receives detailed education about the nature of that disorder and the key components of its clinical management. This process begins during the early phase of intervention. This includes education about the manner in which the disorder is diagnosed, the hypothesised causes, the range of prognosis, both with and without treatment, genetic aspects, and the benefits and risks of specific state-of-the-art biopsychosocial treatment approaches, including coping strategies found beneficial in dealing with acute and persisting symptoms or drug side effects. This education is tailored to the specific experience and features of each person's disorder and lifestyle, and is conducted in a highly interactive way. Furthermore, at least one key family member or close friend is involved in the education process and preferably all members of the household attend. Sessions are held in the home and a supportive counselling approach is adopted rather than a structured didactic presentation. Specially prepared booklets are provided for patients and their carers to read after the sessions and further discussion about issues raised either during the previous sessions or from reading of the booklets is conducted during subsequent sessions.

The aim of this education is primarily to enhance the collaboration between people experiencing mental disorders, and their informal and professional carers. However, we hypothesise that through enhancing understanding of mental disorders in a specific manner, other people in the community become informed of these disorders in a highly personalised way that may assist in their own mental health care. An example may help illustrate this point:

Jackie, a 47-year old widow who lived alone, experienced a severe episode of a panic disorder. She was terrified that something catastrophic would happen if she stayed in her house and sought refuge with her neighbours, who were close friends. They called her family practitioner, who thought that Jackie may have been suffering from an acute episode of schizophrenia. He immediately consulted with the mental health team member who was on duty at his practice. The therapist conducted a brief assessment after perusing the practice notes and considered that the disorder seemed to be a recurrence of previous episodes of acute anxiety that had usually been triggered by stressful life events. Within an hour of the initial call to the family practitioner a meeting was convened by the therapist and team psychiatrist, with Jackie, her neighbour, and another close friend, who lived nearby. During a 90-minute discussion, they were all educated in the key aspects of Jackie's disorder. The key features of a panic disorder were highlighted, a recent stressor that had upset her severely – the threat of being replaced as the church organist – was identified; she had experienced the benefits of relaxing and slowing her breathing to reduce hyperventilation; and was prescribed a sedative tricyclic with explanation of the expected benefits and side effects. Booklets explaining anxiety and its management were left for each person to refer to later. The friends were taught to prompt use of these anxiety management strategies and to assist in monitoring her level of anxiety and sleep. The therapist remained with them for two hours, returning for a further two hours later the same afternoon to reassess progress and to conduct more detailed training in anxiety management with both patient and informal carers. The friends explained that whenever they attempted to reassure Jackie that she would recover and would not become housebound, she became even more anxious. They were taught to avoid reassurance of this kind and to prompt Jackie to chat about topics that were not laden with anxiety.

The following day Jackie was improved and with further intensive treatment had recovered fully within a week. Her neighbour discussed how similar management might help another friend who lived in the village, who appeared to suffer from chronic anxiety symptoms, and was housebound. It was suggested that she ask her friend to discuss the possibility of treatment with her family practitioner. The friend consulted with her doctor, an assessment was made by the practice team and the same therapist began a successful treatment program for another sufferer of an agoraphobic disorder.

During the next year Jackie assisted in the social rehabilitation of two other sufferers of chronic anxiety disorders, one of whom experienced very distressing compulsive thoughts. She took them out with her on shopping trips, and assisted them in attending several church and village functions. This voluntary assistance was made independent of any formal arrangements made by the services and illustrates how an educative approach of this kind tends to facilitate mental health care in the community and to break down the reluctance to seek specialised assistance at an early stage in the development of mental disorders.

Training family practice and mental health staff to conduct reliable assessment of mental disorders

Standardised interview procedures for the assessment of mental disorders are not generally taught in current training programs for family practice or mental health professions. Most modern training programs train generic interviewing skills which emphasise empathy and rapport building supplemented by open-ended questions that may eventually lead to uncovering psychiatric phenomenology. Such a process is seldom the most efficient or the most effective way to conduct a screening for major mental disorders, particularly those characterised by bizarre experience and difficult to explain phenomena, such as delusions, obsessional thoughts, thought interference, or phobic anxiety. Further, the accurate assessment of suicide risk or potential violent behaviour, is seldom achieved without further directed probing.

The past two decades have witnessed the development of several standardised methods for assessment of mental disorders. These methods, while preserving rapport with distressed or disturbed people, seek to clarify the psychopathology that underlies these states. Examples include semi-structured interviews such as the Present State Examination (PSE) (Wing et al, 1974), and the Schedule for Affective Disorder and Schizophrenia (SADS) (Spitzer and Endicott, 1977). Although these interviews were developed to facilitate diagnosis in research studies, their utility in clinical practice provides a reliable method of eliciting and coding the key symptoms of major mental disorders. The PSE and DIS (Diagnostic Interview Schedule: an interview derived from SADS) have both been employed by non-psychiatric interviewers after brief training, with reliability similar to that obtained from psychiatric experts (Wing et al, 1977; Robins et al, 1979).

The PSE was chosen as the standard psychiatric assessment method for the project. Every clinician entering the Buckingham Mental Health Service received training to research reliability standards before they were permitted to assess patients. The self-paced learning program *Detecting the Characteristic Symptoms of Schizophrenia* (Falloon & Lukoff, 1984) was completed prior to workshop training and personal tutoring. Ten audiotaped interviews of people displaying a wide range of phenomenology were then rated and compared with criterion ratings for item to item agreement. A mean level of agreement on the presence and absence of symptoms of 80% was considered to demonstrate competence in this skill. Clinicians also conducted two PSE interviews themselves. These interviews were audiotaped and co-rated by an expert. In addition to meeting the same inter-rater concordance, the quality of interviewing skills were assessed and further training provided where needed. This training ensured that all people engaged in the assessment of people in the service met the minimum standards set for most research projects, and provided valid and reliable psychiatric assessment. It was notable that most of the non-medical staff who undertook this training exceeded the levels of reliability obtained by qualified project psychiatrists (with MRCPsych) after they had completed training. Thus, it was possible to assure the family practitioners that non-medical staff were capable of deputising for trained psychiatrists in the assessment of mental status, at least when assessing routine cases. However, all assessments were reviewed by a psychiatrist, who provided a second assessment where any doubts or discrepancies arose.

For example, a family practitioner sought consultation on a young man, Chris, who had been arrested for making threatening phone calls to a local factory. The doctor was impressed by the bizarre nature of these calls and suspected that this man might be suffering from schizophrenia. Immediately a nurse therapist obtained a detailed history, supplemented with information from the patient's mother, and followed this with a PSE. He consulted with the project psychiatrist upon completion and discussed his findings. Apparently the threatening phone calls always occurred at night after Chris had been drinking heavily with friends. He had a mild learning disability, and was coaxed to make these calls by his drinking companions, who found the behaviour highly amusing. He had no history of mental disorders or evidence of delusions or hallucinations. There was no family history of mental disorders. Chris and his elder brother had both been made redundant from the factory several years earlier and Chris had continued to experience some bitterness about this. It was evident that he had limited interpersonal competence, and was unable to express his frustration in an appropriate manner. His family practitioner received this preliminary feedback and no drugs were prescribed. A follow-up assessment by the team psychiatrist a few days later validated the therapist's assessment, which formed the basis for a report to the court. A program of social skills training was initiated as well as controlled drinking. No further phone calls were made and he began to make friends outside the bar environment. The court placed him on probation on condition that he continued to receive mental health care and abstained from alcohol.

Table 4.1. *Early detection: assessment methods*

	Reference
Stage I: Screening	
10 Question Screening (10 QS)	Falloon 1980
Present State Examination (PSE)	Wing et al 1974
Early Signs Questionnaire (ESQ)	Herz & Melville 1980
Hamilton Rating Scale for Depression	Hamilton 1960
Hamilton Rating Scale for Anxiety	Hamilton 1959
Beck Depression Inventory (BDI)	Beck et al 1961
Mini-mental State Examination	Folstein et al 1975
Eating Attitudes Test (EAT)	Garner et al 1982
Suicide Risk Checklist	Buckingham MHS 1986
Prodromal Signs Checklist	Buckingham MHS 1985
Stage II: Problem analysis	
Problem analysis	Kanfer & Saslow 1965
Target problem rating	Falloon 1985
Family member/carer interview	Falloon et al 1988
Problem solving rating	Falloon et al 1988
Clinical global impressions	Guy 1976
Charing Cross Health Index	Rosser & Kind 1978
Family burden scale	Falloon 1985

In addition to using the full PSE, a number of modules were devised that adapted sections of the PSE for screening for schizophrenic disorders, manic episodes, obsessive-compulsive disorders and depression; the last was combined with the Hamilton Rating Scale for Depression to provide quantitative as well as qualitative ratings. Inter-rater reliability on these subsections was obtained independently. A series of standardised rating scales for eating disorders, and anxiety disorders were deployed after staff training had been completed satisfactorily. The standardised assessments that all therapists are trained to use are summarised in Table 4.1.

While family practitioners are not expected to conduct PSEs, they are trained to detect key features that might indicate the presence of a mental disorder or its prodromal states (Gask et al, 1988; Skuse & Williams, 1984). Ten key symptoms were considered as useful in this screening process:

1 Sleep disturbance
2 Appetite disturbance
3 Changes of energy levels and interests

4 Hopelessness about future prospects
5 Poor concentration
6 Vague or odd speech
7 Worrying about trivial or odd concerns
8 Hearing people talking when nobody about
9 Odd habits involving checking or cleaning
10 Attacks of palpitations, shaking, sweating with fear of heart-attacks or death.

A screening interview, the 10 QS (10-Question Screening), that had been developed for clinical use in the United States, formed the basis for training family practitioners and other professional staff (see Figure 4.2). We planned a series of training seminars for each family practice, but found that attendance was erratic. Instead, family practitioners preferred to meet with mental health therapists individually for case-related discussions and tutorials on a weekly basis. Several family practitioners began employing standardised interviews, such as the Hamilton Rating Scale for Depression and standard assessments for substance abuse, in addition to the 10 QS.

YES NO

- How have you been sleeping in the past week? Any difficulties getting to sleep? Waking early?
- Have you lost your appetite recently? Significant weight loss?
- Any loss of energy or interests recently?
- Have you been worrying a lot about everyday problems?
- Have you had difficulty concentrating on reading or watching television? Been more forgetful than usual?
- How do you see the future? Do you ever feel that life is not worth living? Have you ever felt you would like to end it all?
- Have you any odd habits, like checking or cleaning more than other people?
- Do you ever have attacks of palpitations, sweating, shaking or dizziness with feelings of intense fear?
- Has anybody commented that your speech has become odd or difficult to understand?
- Have you ever had the experience of hearing peoples' voices when nobody seems to be around?

Figure 4.2. The 10 Question Screening (10 QS) for mental health assessment in primary health care.

Despite the lack of formality of this training it was apparent that the family practitioners enhanced their skills at detecting possible cases of serious mental disorders considerably. Regular discussions with psychiatrists occurred, both during practice meetings, and at regular family practice training and liaison meetings, where the psychiatrists were welcomed as 'honorary family practitioners'. The opportunity for this mutual training was a benefit of the integrated service approach.

One problem that resulted from this training was that a few family practitioners employed the easy access to specialist assessment as a means of screening a large proportion of people who presented to them in a distressed state. They tended to invite therapists to provide management for everyone with minor stress who consulted with them, even when it was clear that the stress responses were far removed from any form of mental disorder. They failed to attempt to conduct any preliminary screening themselves, stating that they were too busy, or that they had not been adequately trained to carry out this activity (despite constant efforts of mental health therapists to provide such training). This posed a difficult dilemma. We did not want to discourage the specific family practitioners from asking for second opinions about many of these cases, merely to screen in a slightly more conservative fashion. However, this proved extremely difficult, and the only answer we were able to achieve was that we agreed to assess those referred upon demand, but to ensure that immediate feedback was provided to the family practitioner about cases where screening was grossly inappropriate. Such patients were returned immediately to the management of the family practitioner, accompanied by any useful guidelines about how we might have managed the case. However, this excessive zeal for utilising mental health consultation was balanced by a few family practitioners who made little use of our expertise. Fortunately these practitioners appeared very competent in the assessment and clinical management of most mental disorders, combining drugs and counselling methods in an effective manner.

A similar individually tailored approach was applied to training non-psychiatric nurses, such as health visitors and district nurses. Here a major impediment to learning simple diagnostic screening methods was previous training in counselling methods. Most community nurses had been advised that under no circumstances should they ask their patients any direct questions about their mental states.

Instead they were told that patients would self-disclose details such as their plans for suicide, compulsive thoughts and behaviours, or experiences of hallucinations, providing they maintained empathic rapport throughout their contact. Furthermore they were imbued with a concern for confidentiality, that made it impossible for them to consider interviewing a spouse or parent of a patient, for fear of damaging their confiding relationship with the index patient. Such attitudes proved very rigid and were only shaken when these community nurses participated in joint assessment interviews with mental health therapists.

Special topics: suicide risk and schizophrenia

Two areas where early intervention is a major goal are in detecting people at risk for suicide and those showing the early signs of schizophrenia. Both these problems have a low frequency of occurrence. The ability to forestall suicide attempts and their resulting fatalities has been suggested as an indication of the success of a community-based mental health service (Renvoize & Clayden, 1990). The ability to minimise the morbidity of schizophrenic disorders is another index of an effective service. Despite their low frequency, both present major public health problems in industrialised countries and are the chief source of admissions to the costly intensive treatment services traditionally provided in hospitals. The challenge these problems present tends to be one key concern for those planning services for communities. It is a challenge that must be met.

Family practitioners and mental health therapists were alerted to the possibility that any person suffering from a major mental disorder, particularly depressive episodes, schizophrenia or severe persistent anxiety states may have a high risk of suicide. In addition, alcoholism and major stress, especially bereavement and marital breakdown where loss is profound, carry a similarly increased risk. Reliable methods of determining this risk have yet to be formulated, and current studies have shown how difficult it is to predict the specific individuals who will commit suicide (Hawton & Catalan, 1987). Nevertheless a review of the literature enabled us to devise a checklist of background and clinical risk factors (see Table 4.2).

Whenever a person was suspected of having thoughts of suicide or

Table 4.2. *Assessment of suicide risk factors*

Male
Living alone
Single/separated/divorced/widowed
Unemployed
Recent major stress (especially loss)
Alcohol or drug abuse
Major mental illness
Serious physical illness
Profound, persistent hopelessness
Extreme frustration
Previous suicide attempt

self-destruction family practitioners were asked to consult immediately. Therapists conducted a tactful and comprehensive screening that aims to develop rapport and trust, while displaying concern about current life problems. The assessment enables the checklist to be completed. If six or more items are checked as present, and the person is currently actively contemplating suicide, the suicide risk is considered 'high'. This triggers a program of intensive suicide management that is described in detail in Chapter 6.

Detection of schizophrenia at an early phase and the instigation of effective management is probably the best way to reduce the risk of a chronic disabling course (Crow et al, 1986). Special efforts were made to devise a program which facilitated early recognition of schizophrenia, based on recent research indicating that most episodes of schizophrenia, including the initial episodes, begin after a period of prodromal symptoms, usually lasting several weeks or months (Herz & Melville, 1980; Docherty et al, 1978; Birchwood et al, 1989).

A two-stage approach has been developed, entailing (1) training family practitioners to recognise prodromal symptoms and, without delay, to refer such people for (2) immediate specialised mental health assessment.

Family practitioner assessment of prodromal signs of schizophrenia

All family practitioners were trained to recognise eight features that might indicate the early stage of an episode of schizophrenia. These

Table 4.3. *Prodromal signs checklist*

Onset of one of the following without explanation
Marked peculiar behaviour
Inappropriate, or loss of, expression of feelings
Speech that is difficult to follow
Marked lack of speech and thoughts
Marked preoccupation with odd ideas
Ideas of reference – things have special meanings
Persistent feelings of unreality
Changes in the way things appear, sound or smell

Source: From DSM-III, 1980.

symptoms are listed in Table 4.3. They are derived from the
prodromal signs outlined in DSM III-R. A checklist that included
brief elaboration of these features was provided for the family
practitioners to refer to whenever they suspected a possible case.
Training has been conducted on an individual consultation basis for
half the family practitioners and in group seminars for the remainder. Role playing of examples of the prodromal symptoms was used
to clarify their nature. Most family practitioners reported that they
readily recognise these features when they occur, but had usually
hesitated to go to the trouble to refer such cases to a mental health
clinic unless they became much worse. The close collaboration with
the mental health service in this project facilitated informal consultation, and the family practitioners gave assurances that any person
with any unusual features would be referred for further assessment
without delay.

Assessment of prodromal states by mental health professionals

The availability of 24-hour assessment by a multidisciplinary team
of mental health professionals, including a senior psychiatrist,
ensures that assessment can be made within an hour of referral,
usually within a few minutes of the request. The mental health
assessment includes:

(*a*) Patient and key caregiver (usually a relative or household
member) completes the modified version of the Early Signs Questionnaire (ESQ; Herz & Melville, 1980). This lists features found in the
prodromes of florid schizophrenic episodes, and is used to prompt
patients and their caregivers to specify prodromal symptoms.

(*b*) If features reported by the family practitioner or noted on the ESQ suggest a prodromal state, a trained mental health professional completes a Present State Examination.

(*c*) A psychiatric, medical, drug and family history is obtained using the systematic schedule developed for the project. Substance abuse and organic medical conditions that may have contributed to the current state are excluded by history and examination, supervised by the family practitioner and psychiatrist. People with first-degree relatives who have suffered schizophrenia; those with severe unremitting stressors; those who have had prodromal episodes in the past; and those who have made unexplained suicide attempts are all considered to have a higher risk of schizophrenia than the average person living in the community.

(*d*) The differential psychiatric diagnosis is considered in consultation with a psychiatrist. This includes consideration that the prodromal features could be the early stage of a manic episode, atypical depression or acute anxiety disorder. A history of previous episodes of mental disorders and family history provide additional information to assist in defining the probability that the current state represents the initial phase of a first episode of a schizophrenic psychosis. In all such cases a project psychiatrist conducts an independent assessment to validate key aspects of the mental health assessment, usually on the day the person presents with the features at the family practice.

Once it has been established that a person is suspected of experiencing a prodrome of schizophrenia an integrated programme of crisis management is initiated without delay. This includes education, stress management and neuroleptic medication. Each component is targeted according to individual needs within a structured clinical management protocol.

These two examples of clinical management of suicide risk and early detection of schizophrenia demonstrate the careful way in which procedures are developed within the integrated service to ensure that all potentially disabling disorders are managed in a consistent manner, that aims to ensure that people receive the optimal treatment in the most efficient manner. Early signs of anxiety, depression, abnormal eating behaviour, and serious psychosocial disturbance are managed according to similar standardised procedures.

It may be evident that substantial efforts have been made to define mental disorders. The key reason for this is that this mental health service, in common with most in the UK, was contracted to provide services for people experiencing mental disorders. People with difficulty and distress that do not meet the criteria for the diagnosis of a mental disorder are not the primary target population for these services. We consider that the management of people with features suggesting that they may be in the early phases of mental disorders, or who are considered to have a very high risk of developing one, is a legitimate extension of this contract. However, it seems important not to attempt to provide mental health treatment for those people for whom other agencies, such as social services, housing, financial and occupational, could provide the primary resolution for their problems and the associated distress. In these cases, after completing the screening assessments, people are assisted to obtain consultation from those appropriate agencies. At times this involves considerable advocacy from the mental health therapists and family practitioners, even at times leading to local campaigns for the provision of adequate services. The service always takes a strong stand on ensuring that its primary role is that of a *health agency, not a social agency,* and the community is reminded of the dangers in confusing these roles, particularly where this leads to the inappropriate use of medical treatments for the suppression of social deviance.

Conclusion

The early detection of mental disorders in the community involves a two-stage process, with informal screening by family practitioners coupled by readily accessible mental health assessment using structured rating scales and diagnostic instruments. Figure 4.1 summarises this process. To this point the emphasis has been on detection of psychiatric syndromes or prodromes. Once the psychiatric classification has been clarified and the priority of care established, further assessment efforts are focussed on the functional problems that are associated with the disorder, both those that have contributed to the onset of the current episode and its maintenance, as well as those factors that may make the person more vulnerable to subsequent episodes. These issues will be dealt with in the next chapter.

References

Beck A.T., Ward C.H., Mendelsohn M., Mock J. & Erbaugh J. (1961) An inventory for measuring depression. *Archives of General Psychiatry,* **4**, 561–571.

Birchwood M., Smith J.V.E. & Macmillan J.F. (1989) The development and implementation of an early warning system to control relapse in schizophrenia. *Psychological Medicine,* **19**, 649–656.

Brodaty H. & Andrews G. (1983) Brief psychotherapy in family practice: a controlled prospective intervention trial. *British Journal of Psychiatry,* **143**, 11–19.

Crow T.J., MacMillan J.F., Johnson A.L. & Johnstone E.C. (1986) A randomised controlled trial of prophylactic neuroleptic treatment. *British Journal of Psychiatry,* **148**, 120–127.

Dilling H. & Weyrerer S. (1984) Prevalence of mental disorders in the small town rural region of Traunstein (Upper Bavaria). *Acta Psychiatrica Scandinavica,* **69**, 60–79

Docherty J.P., van Kammen D.P. & Siris S.G. (1978) Stages of schizophrenic psychosis. *American Journal of Psychiatry,* **135**, 420–426.

Falloon I.R.H. (1985) *Family management of schizophrenia.* Johns Hopkins University Press, Baltimore.

Falloon I.R.H. & Lukoff D. (1984) *Schizophrenia: Interview strategies for detecting characteristic symptoms.* Guilford Press, New York.

Falloon I., Mueser K., Gingerich S., Rappaport S., McGill C. & Hole V. (1988) *Behavioural family therapy: a workbook.* Buckingham Mental Health Service, Buckingham.

Folstein M.F., Folstein S.E. & McHugh P.R. (1975) 'Mini-Mental State': a practical method for grading the cognitive state of patients for the clinician. *Journal of Psychiatric Research,* **12**, 189–198.

Garner D.M., Olmstead M.P., Bohr Y. & Garfinkel P.E. (1982) The Eating Attitudes Test: psychometric features and clinical correlates. *Psychological Medicine,* **12**, 871–878.

Gask L., Goldberg D.P., Lesser A. & Miller T. (1988) Improving the psychiatric skills of the general practice trainee. *Medical Education,* **22**, 132–138.

Goldberg D.P. & Huxley P. (1980) *Mental illness in the community: The pathway to psychiatric care.* Tavistock, London.

Guy W. (1976) *E.C.D.E.U. Assessment manual for psychopharmacology.* U.S. Department of Health, Education and Welfare, Washington, D.C.

Hamilton M. (1959) The assessment of anxiety states by rating. *British Journal of Medical Psychology,* **32**, 50–58.

Hamilton M. (1960) A rating scale for depression. *Journal of Neurology Neurosurgery & Psychiatry,* **23**, 56–62.

Hawton K. & Catalan J. (1987) *Attempted suicide: a practical guide to its nature and management,* 2nd edn. Oxford University Press, Oxford.

Herz M.I. & Melville C. (1980) Relapse in schizophrenia. *American Journal of Psychiatry*, **137**, 801–805.

Kanfer F.H. & Saslow G. (1965) Behavioral analysis: an alternative to diagnostic classification. *Archives of General Psychiatry*, **12**, 529–538.

Renvoize E. & Clayden D. (1990) Can suicide rate be used as a performance indicator in mental illness? *Health Trends*, **12**, 16–19.

Robins L., Helzer J., Croughan J., Williams J.B.W. & Spitzer R.L. (1979) *The NIMH Diagnostic Interview Schedule (DIS)*, Version II. National Institute of Mental Health, Washington, D.C.

Rosser R.M. & Kind P. (1978) A scale of valuations of states of illness: Is there a social consensus? *International Journal of Epidemiology*, **7**, 347–358.

Skuse D. & Williams P. (1984) Screening for psychiatric disorder. *Psychological Medicine*, **14**, 365–378.

Spitzer, R.L. & Endicott, J. (1977) *Schedule for affective disorders and schizophrenia*. Columbia University, New York.

Wing, J.K., Cooper, J.E. & Sartorius, N. (1974) *Measurement and classification of psychiatric symptoms*. Cambridge University Press, Cambridge.

Wing J.K., Nixon J.M., Mann S.A. & Leff J.P. (1977) Reliability of the PSE used in a population survey. *Psychological Medicine*, **7**, 505–516.

5

Problem-based assessment of functioning

In this chapter we describe the more detailed problem-based assessment employed in integrated mental health care after the initial screening assessment has been completed. This functional assessment takes us beyond establishing the mere diagnosis of a person's disorder and seeks to establish the exact nature of the problems that prevent them from achieving their expected level of everyday functioning. Furthermore, it assists the therapist in formulating the most efficient intervention strategies to minimise this disability and restore expected functioning. As well as achieving short term resolution of the specific features associated with the direct manifestations of the disorder, problems that may increase the risk of further recurrences, or delay full recovery may be targeted for intervention. The functional assessment consists of the following main components (see Appendix 2):

1 Screening for problems that may contribute to continuing vulnerability and stress.
2 Analysis of key current problems.
3 Setting goals for intervention.
4 Formulating intervention strategies.
5 Devising methods for monitoring progress towards therapeutic goals.

Screening for persisting risk factors

In Chapter 4 we described the background information obtained during the preliminary screening process. Further details are then obtained that may help tailor the intervention programme to each

Table 5.1. *Early detection strategies*

Vulnerability factors
Genetic; family history
Obstetric complications
Epilepsy; neurological signs
Lower IQ than expected

Provoking factors
Post-natal
Substance misuse; stimulants
Major life stress/poor coping capacity

Enhanced screening
Improved public awareness
Primary care screening
Standardised mental health assessment
Recognition of prodromal states

person's profile of vulnerability to current and future episodes of a disorder. A checklist is used to ensure that key information is obtained (see Table 5.1). This is based upon research findings on the long-term outcome of mental disorders (Brown & Harris, 1978; Leff & Vaughn, 1985; Nuechterlein, 1990). This same assessment forms part of the efforts (outlined in Chapter 7) to minimise the risk of future episodes. However, as the presence of factors such as high environmental stress levels, or persisting drug taking frequently play a part in determining the success of early intervention, these are often targeted for immediate intervention.

In addition to obtaining further details of background deficits, the therapist notes any potential assets that may be employed to any key problems. These may include material assets such as housing, finances, employment, personal transport, as well as education, job training, problem-solving skills, social skills and supportive social networks.

Problem analysis

The aim of the problem analysis is to pinpoint one or two key problems that appear closely linked with the main areas of disability associated with the mental disorder, and to determine the most efficient way of resolving these problems. This is achieved through the following steps:

1 Pinpointing the problem.
2 Defining the immediate antecedents and consequences of the problem.
3 Defining the factors that modify the severity of the problem.
4 Determining motivation to resolve the problem.
5 Outlining all current efforts to resolve the problem.

Pinpointing the problem

The initial step is undoubtedly the most important and most difficult. This entails defining the one or two key problems associated with the impairment of the mental disorder. In some cases these may be directly related to the disorder; for example, a person with an agoraphobic disorder may see their key problem as coping with panic attacks. In other cases the problem may only be defined after careful interviewing, such as the woman with agoraphobia, who had a jealous husband who preferred to have his wife stay in the safety of the home, and who repeatedly sabotaged her efforts to overcome her anxieties. In complex cases such as this the therapist takes a detective role, and attempts to pinpoint the key issue that may underlie the failure of repeated efforts to overcome impairments. As we have discussed above, the disorder may not remit where persisting serious stresses continue to fuel the fire, and these stresses may need to be defined, prioritised and reduced before any direct efforts to modify anxiety, depression or thought disturbance are likely to prove effective.

The aim is always to pinpoint the key issue that can be most readily addressed, and efficiently resolved, resulting in maximal improvement for minimal cost to the sufferer, social network and professional resources. This cognitive-behavioural approach contrasts with most other mental health approaches in that it seeks to employ the most straightforward method of minimising disability. Problem resolution usually employs a brainstorming approach that enables biological, psychological and social factors to be considered fully in all aspects of assessment and treatment. Wherever possible attempts are made to ensure that long-term reductions in disability are achieved, and not merely short-term symptom suppression.

Unravelling intertwined problem issues is seldom achieved in one session, and this assessment may be extended over several sessions. Of course, during this time immediate steps may have to be taken to relieve current suffering. Taking adequate time to define problem issues in this manner may appear a luxury that few services can afford, but where problems are targeted in this way the solutions may be relatively straightforward, and are more likely to succeed in providing lasting benefits. An hour or two of careful problem analysis may save months of frustrating application of poorly understood, ineffective intervention strategies. It also ensures that the treatment is tailored to the needs of the individual, and is therefore more likely to be acceptable to that person and to produce the desired results. Too often in recent times mental health professionals have strayed away from the true spirit of behavioural analysis (see Kanfer & Saslow, 1965) where clinical management is linked directly to individual assessment of needs. Instead, people are offered 'packages' of treatment, many elements of which may have little relevance for them or their real difficulties.

Once the problem has been pinpointed it is described in detail using everyday language. In addition, a brief history of the development of the problem may be provided.

Determining the antecedents and consequences

All circumstances in which the problem seems to emerge are specified, particularly those specific circumstances that immediately precede the problem; e.g. sequence of events preceding a violent outburst, panic attack, suicidal thought, auditory hallucination, etc. Patterns may emerge from this assessment. For example, a young woman noted that she heard voices most frequently when walking in the street, shopping in a supermarket, and attending a wedding. It transpired that all these events involved crowded places, and were made even worse when she was tired, and within two days of her menstrual period.

Such antecedents are seldom as consistent as the above example, and it is important that the assessor does not prejudge the assessment to fit existing notions about certain disorders. The assessor may choose to give the person a diary to monitor occurrence of a clearly defined problem. In addition to defining the frequency, and/ or severity of the problem, the record may include a brief description of the context in which the problem occurs. Where reliable self-monitoring is not feasible, a carer may assist, or in rare instances a professional may be employed to monitor the problem in this manner.

All responses that occur immediately after the problem emerges are similarly specified. Operant conditioning principles suggest that the immediate responses to an event may increase or decrease the likelihood of the event recurring. Such a principle may be used to increase desirable events by providing specific pleasant responses as immediate consequences of specific events. On the other hand undesirable events are less likely to occur where they do not receive any immediate pleasing consequences. The problem analysis seeks to define the various consequences of problems so that any patterns of response that may be contributing (often unwittingly) to increased occurrence of the problem can be recognised and remedied. The use of reassurance is a common example of unwitting reinforcement of statements about depressive moods or unpleasant thoughts and plays a key role in the maintenance of persisting obsessional and dysthymic states.

An example of this analysis of contingencies surrounding a problem behaviour was a young woman, Phyllis, who had an eating disorder. Her bingeing was preceded by the following:

feeling hungry
worrying about work
fear her boyfriend would leave her
returning home at any time
feeling bored
being at home alone

Once she began bingeing the following consequences occurred:

she felt relaxed
her boyfriend became concerned
she felt more energetic and initiated activity

Despite the fact that about half an hour after the binge she began worrying about her weight gain, the food intake appeared to have immediate anxiety-reducing effect which enhanced the likelihood that it would recur. The immediate short-term pleasant effect outweighed the longer-term undesired effect. Thus, a strategy to modify this pattern of response might aim to change the triggers and/or the rewards associated with bingeing. This might include developing alternative ways of coping with the circumstances that tend to trigger the unwanted behaviour.

Frequency and intensity of the problem

The frequency and intensity of a particular problem may have a major bearing on the disability that it is likely to cause. People are instructed to estimate the severity of the problem in these terms. This may prove difficult, particularly where the frequency and intensity varies widely on a day-to-day basis. In such cases it may help to request the person to chart each time the problem occurs and its maximum intensity at that time. Where the problem is persistent, such as a depressed mood, the person may record its intensity at predetermined times during the day, usually on the hour.

Modifying factors

The therapist enquires about all circumstances that appear to make the problem better or worse. This information may provide clues to strategies that might be employed in the management plan to minimise the severity of a problem. It is always wise to make use of strategies which people are already employing themselves or which are partly effective as these are easier to develop and are more likely to be acceptable to the person. In the case of the bingeing problem described above the following modifying factors may have played a part.

Factors that might make the problem better:

somebody at home with me
affection from my boyfriend, even a phone call if he's unable to visit
my boss showing appreciation at work
getting involved in some constructive activity or reading

Factors that might make the problem worse:

feeling tired
having a bad day at work
two days before menstrual period

boyfriend away on business trip

Some of these modifying factors may seem similar to the antecedents. It is not essential that a distinction is made between these. A *trigger* tends to be something that happens immediately before the event, whereas a *modifying factor* tends to be a more general state that makes a person more susceptible to the problem occurring.

Gains and losses from problem resolution

The resolution of a problem usually leads to improvements of everyday functioning, but in our far from perfect world there are also usually some drawbacks to contend with. The loss of the support provided for the role of a 'sick' person is a typical example of this. Where chronic disabling problems have been resolved for people, considerable readjustment may be needed to a lifestyle that has been carefully tailored to cope with the disability. This is clearly seen in persons who are moving from institutional care to community living settings, many of whom view the expected gains as less than the potential benefits, and are consequently lacking in motivation for change that others view with enthusiasm. Similar losses are found in all problems, and may explain why many people who have all the strategies and skills to overcome their problems themselves, still fail to make progress. Thus, while the gains from problem resolution are usually quite clear, the losses may be more subtle, yet crucial to efficient intervention. In the example we have been considering, the relevant gains and losses included:

Expected gains:

> less worry about food and weight
> more money
> feeling more in control of my life

Expected losses:

> more effort needed to do constructive things
> boyfriend might not be so considerate

Current problem-solving efforts

A basic principle of cognitive-behavioural psychology is that people are always doing their very best to resolve each and every problem.

The strategies they employ may at times appear self-defeating to the objective observer, but at the time they are deployed, they represent that person's best attempted solution. At other times the strategies people use are fully or partially successful, and may resemble closely the therapeutic procedures that we might plan to offer. A skilled therapist is able to uncover the specific self-help skills each person employs to cope with their specific problems. The therapist can then build on strategies that already exist in the person's repertoire, shaping and refining them so that they provide more consistent benefits. This helps develop a close working relationship between the person and their therapist, where that individual's skills and coping efforts are clearly validated.

When her therapist enquired about the ways in which Phyllis currently attempted to deal with her bingeing problem, she reported the following:

> tell myself not to
> phone my boyfriend
> asked advice from a close friend
> went to my family doctor
> avoid buying food treats
> arrange for boyfriend to take me home after work
> distract myself; try to do some chore that needs doing to keep busy
> just give in to urge without worrying

It is clear that this person had a wide range of self-help strategies, all of which helped to a limited extent. Like most people, her problem was not present continuously, so that for most of the time her efforts were controlling it in a highly effective manner. The therapist's task then became one of assisting Phyllis to apply her coping strategies more efficiently at specific times, rather than merely teaching her strategies from scratch. Even a therapist with limited experience at treating a person suffering an eating disorder can apply commonsense and develop an effective therapeutic plan from this information.

In addition to specific problem solving, the therapist is invited to summarise general assets and deficits the individual and their social network possess in their problem-solving functions. These may include factors such as education, social support systems, past experience, finances, help-seeking and interpersonal skills, attitudes towards adversity, cultural factors, persisting stresses, etc. One of the commonest issues concerns people who have difficulty transferring skills they use in one setting to another. For example, many people who display excellent problem-solving skills in the workplace are unable to deploy the same management skills in their family settings. In such cases the therapist merely has to facilitate effective transfer of skills from one situation to another to enhance problem resolution.

Much concern is often expressed about problems therapists encounter when working with people from cultural backgrounds that differ markedly from their own. This approach to functional analysis reduces such problems by considering coping patterns within each individual's social support system. Where patterns of coping responses are viewed as appropriate and effective within a cultural group the therapists are expected to endorse them and facilitate their consistent use, no matter how deviant the responses may appear to them, providing of course that the behaviour remains within the constraints of the laws of the community. Where the coping responses of one person conflict with the cultural values of their immediate support network, this is likely to produce added stress and consequently impair the effectiveness of the coping strategy for that person. The therapist is expected to assist the individual to resolve such conflicts, either by helping to develop alternative strategies that are more readily supported by the cultural group, or by addressing directly that person's conflicts with his or her support network. The choice between these options will be made primarily by the distressed individual.

Reinforcement survey

This is a survey of everyday lifestyle. It provides specific information about how a person spends his/her time, or at least their perception of how they spend their time. In addition, the therapist is able to see those areas where a person's actual everyday activities fall short of their expected and desired lifestyle. This provides a useful guide to the subjective quality of life of each person. Where current activities approximate desired activities, regardless of the person's lifestyle, it may be assumed that the person considers that they are leading the kind of life that they wish, and have little motivation to change, even when the therapist may consider that many improvements may be feasible. On the other hand, where a person becomes resigned to a deprived lifestyle, merely because they cannot see any way of achieving their desired improvements (a) because they have not sampled enough activities to be aware of the choices open to them; or (b) because of continued impairment or disability from their mental disorders. In these situations the reinforcement survey may prompt a reassessment of current circumstances, particularly if tangible assistance is being promised by the therapist and the goals appear realistic.

Persons are asked to list all current activities, people, places and material objects with which they spend most of their time. The precise amounts of time are not assessed (self-reporting of such details is seldom accurate). There may be considerable overlap between the different sections. For example, a person may spend considerable time in the family lounge, often accompanied by another household member, watching the television (the latter being a material object). A person who spends much time at work in an office may report spending most of their time with particular workmates and with a specific piece of equipment, such as a typewriter or word-processor. Apart from the distortions that are inherent in self-reports from people who are unimpaired by mental disorders, therapists need to remember that the perceptions of persons suffering from disabling mental disorders of their daily lives may be further distorted. For example, a depressed person may tend to focus on unpleasant activities and not report constructive activities; someone with an eating disorder may distort the time spent engaged in eating behaviours, and a person in a manic state may overemphasise accomplishments. People in depressive and obsessional states may have a tendency to have high expectations of what they would rather be doing with their time and express regret that their achievements are minimal.

A further aspect of the survey of reinforcements involves asking the person to list all major sources of displeasure to which he or she is exposed, or actively avoids. In some cases these aversive situations may be a temporary effect associated with their current disabilities, but in others, impairments, such as persisting anxiety may have led to a very restricted lifestyle. The potential for reducing the severity of such disability may enable such persons to consider restoration of a former, more fulfilling lifestyle.

It is evident that a very straightforward discussion of how people spend their time may provide substantial assistance in defining rehabilitative goals. In addition, it may assist the therapist to target specific everyday activities, people, places and objects that could facilitate change through their potential for positive reinforcement.

Where a more detailed lifestyle survey is required, particularly in the rehabilitation of handicapped individuals, standardised measures of the quality of life may be added to this assessment.

Setting personal goals

The functional relevance of a person's problems depends ultimately on how they impede progress towards each person's goals of everyday life. Although many people will not conceptualise their everyday lives in terms of goal achievement, they nonetheless will readily recognise when a problem disrupts and limits their functioning no matter how routine and mundane that appears. The aim of our approach is to enhance the quality of life of persons suffering directly and indirectly (e.g. carers, friends) from the effects of mental disorders. For this reason it is essential that therapy targets not merely the disorder directly, but also ensures that people are able to continue to exploit their abilities to maintain and enhance their everyday lifestyles. This is particularly important where disability persists despite the best therapeutic interventions. However, it is also relevant to those people with mild disability, who may experience a breakdown in their work, leisure, social and personal relationships as a result of the disruption caused by relatively mild disorders, or occasionally as a result of the treatment they receive.

Goal setting includes the following steps:

pinpoint the goal exactly
ensure that it is readily achievable, and will lead to improved quality of life for the person
determine those steps already achieved
outline problems needed to be overcome to achieve goal
note support and conflict in the immediate social network that may affect goal achievement
rehearse with the person strategies for dealing with the difficulties that may arise in working towards the goal

Using this approach, the person is invited to outline one or two goals that they would like to achieve within the next three to six months (depending on the expected duration of the intervention program), on the assumption that their current problems can be resolved or reduced. Readily achievable everyday goals that will make small, but significant improvements in the person's quality of life are encouraged, rather than major achievements or goals that may have little long-term impact on the person's everyday functioning. Thus, a goal to get a part-time job may be considered more beneficial than an annual holiday at a beach resort; or starting a further education class more realistic than entering an extremely challenging training course.

Many persons, who are severely disabled at the time of this interview, or who have devoted much of their efforts to coping with long-term disabilities, may have difficulty considering life-change goals. They may be assisted by recalling the discrepancies they cited between their current and desired levels of functioning in the reinforcement survey. The therapist may further help by encouraging them to break down long range objectives into a series of intermediate steps. Although the ultimate goal may be unattainable at this time, initial steps towards that goal may be feasible objectives. One person, who was eager to move out of her parents' home, get married and start a family, was able to break down these objectives to initial goals of cooking the family dinner every Thursday, and joining an art club, where she hoped she could meet people of both sexes and enhance her skills at developing close friendships.

The goals set are the personal aims of each person, and should not be targeted specifically to change another person's behaviour. For example, the goals of 'getting Sam better' or 'my wife becoming more affectionate towards me' are avoided. Such goals may be major obstacles preventing those people achieving the changes they desire in their own lives, and may often need to be resolved before significant progress can be achieved.

Each goal is defined in a precise manner that permits all people involved in the therapy to recognise clearly the goal and subsequently to acknowledge its achievement. The following examples compare initial goal statements with final definitions refined with the assistance of the therapist:

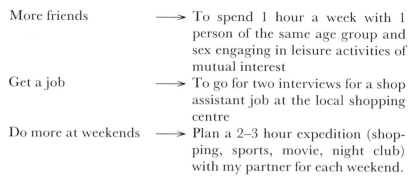

More friends   ⟶ To spend 1 hour a week with 1 person of the same age group and sex engaging in leisure activities of mutual interest

Get a job   ⟶ To go for two interviews for a shop assistant job at the local shopping centre

Do more at weekends   ⟶ Plan a 2–3 hour expedition (shopping, sports, movie, night club) with my partner for each weekend.

Once a person's goals have been pinpointed, all steps that they have already taken towards achieving these goals are listed. These may include concrete steps, such as saving money to pay the fees of a course, or less tangible steps, such as making a definite commitment to pursue the goal. Expected major obstacles to overcome are outlined briefly, in addition to the levels of support for work on each goal that are anticipated from friends and family.

This goal setting process provides the therapist with a clear understanding of the motivation of each person to make changes in their lives. Occasionally people may state that they are fully content, and that they have no desire to change their lifestyles in any way at all. However, this situation is rare. Moreover, many people with severe disabilities who have been considered to lack motivation and drive, emerge eager to initiate changes in their lives after their needs have been addressed in this manner. One person said he was so delighted that after so many years somebody actually invited him to choose his own goals rather than tell him what they thought he should be doing. Inevitably, some people have extreme difficulty setting personal goals, and for some who are very disabled this process may take several hours over several sessions. Whilst the therapist attempts to remain a neutral facilitator at all times, prompted suggestions and supportive feedback may help disabled to consider some of the possible goals he or she might choose.

Development of a problem management plan

The final component of the comprehensive assessment entails the development of the problem management plan. If the initial problem analysis has been completed in a careful fashion, and the therapist is trained in state-of-the-art intervention strategies, this task will usually fall into place. The following steps are undertaken:

    select the key problem for initial intervention
    define the method to be used to monitor progress
    assess baseline level of severity of the problem
    define the aim of the clinical management plan
    devise a detailed intervention strategy

Where more than one problem has been assessed, it is necessary to decide which problem will be addressed first. This decision is made on the basis of the problem that, when resolved, is likely to produce the most benefits for the person and his/her social network, in terms of personal goals as well as relief of distress. At times it may be formulated that resolution of one problem may contribute to full or partial resolution of the other. Regardless, it is usually advisable to tackle one problem at a time, so that the specific benefits of each intervention plan can be evaluated in turn.

Monitoring progress

The therapist chooses a straightforward method of rating change in the severity of the problem that will provide an accurate reflection of progress. On occasions this may be the total score on a standardised rating scale (e.g. Hamilton Depression Scales), but more often one specific item from a scale will be targeted for rating. For example, if a person's targeted problem is that of getting off to sleep at night, the rating scale item that deals with that specific problem will be a more accurate reflection of progress than a total score of 18 items that deal with a wide range of problems associated with depressive disorders.

Many targeted problems are highly specific, and the therapist may construct a scale that is specifically targeted to that person's problems. A generic scale with severity ratings from 0 = no problem to 8 = maximum severity may be personalised in this manner. Examples of these are:

Sleep problem ⟶ Difficulty getting to sleep when going to bed after 10.30 at night (0 = getting to sleep within 30 min, 2 = getting to sleep within 60 min. 4 = getting to sleep within 90 min, 6 = getting to sleep within 120 min, 8 = not getting to sleep in 180 min)

Note that the odd numbers on the scale are not assigned values, but can be used to reflect intermediate ratings. For example a rating of 1 would indicate getting to sleep in around 45 minutes.

Concentration problem ⟶ Difficulty reading or watching television, with thoughts wandering to worries about minor problems (0 = reading or watching TV for 60 min without major disruption in thoughts, 2 = reading or watching TV for 45 min, 4 = reading or watching TV for 30 min, 6 = reading or watching TV for 15 min, 8 = reading or watching TV for less than 5 min)

Anxiety problem ⟶ Experiencing a panic attack with sweating, shaking, heart pounding, feeling faint, and thoughts of going crazy (0 = no panics in past 5 days, 2 = 2 panics in past 5 days, 4 = 4 panics in past 5 days, 6 = 6 panics in past 5 days, 8 = 8 or more panics in past 5 days)

Each of these scales is made to fit the person's current situation, and the ratings are defined clearly. For clinical purposes it is not essential to standardise these ratings in terms of their psychometric properties. They simply provide a clear chart of that person's progress that can be readily shared with sufferers and carers as well as all professional members of the service (see Figure 5.1).

Ratings of the severity of each problem in the week or two before therapeutic interventions are initiated provide a baseline of the course of the problem during a period when the person and carers are applying their best efforts to resolve the problem. Effective professional intervention will be reflected in reduction in the severity of the ratings during the period it is applied. Structuring therapeutic inputs in this way provides a clearer guide to the efficacy of treatment approaches, and assists in the review process of each case. More complex multiple-baseline designs can enable scientist-practitioners to develop new therapeutic strategies within clinical

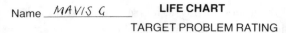

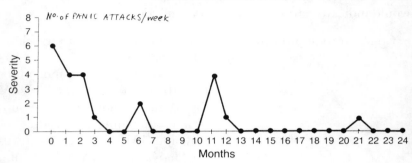

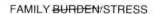

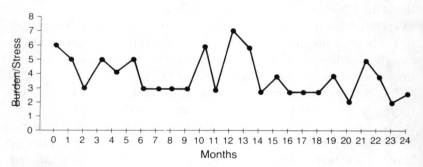

Figure 5.1. Life chart of progress on clinical, social and carer problems.

practice. Such methods are beyond the scope of this book, but are well reviewed in several publications (Barlow et al, 1984; Shapiro, 1961).

Intervention plans

The details of the intervention plan are outlined step-by-step. The exact methods that will be used and the duration of initial applications are listed. Any modifications from validated procedures are noted. Any major hitches that can be anticipated are noted, along with strategies that will be applied to deal with them. For example, a neuroleptic drug may have a high risk of producing specific unwanted effects at the dosage used. Remedies for coping with such effects are planned in anticipation, not when a crisis arises. Similarly, where assessment suggests that poor adherence to a therapeutic plan is likely, strategies are designed to enhance compliance from the initial phase of the program. An example of a comprehensive intervention plan for a person who has a targeted problem of getting off to sleep within 30 minutes is provided:

1 Educate person and partner about coping with sleep disturbance: 1 session.
2 Recommend reduced caffeine intake to two cups of coffee daily.
3 Progressive muscular relaxation training (PMR): 2 sessions.
4 Problem solving training may be needed if PMR fails to reduce worrying thoughts: 1 session + follow-up session.
5 Educate family doctor about benefits and risks of short-acting hypnotic drugs (person stopped taking them after terrifying nightmares).
6 Review in two weeks at family practice meeting.

You will note that a time and venue for an interim review of the effectiveness of the plan is included. The example provided here was a person who subsequently developed a depressive episode. However, the early intervention with a problem-based approach may have limited the disability, and enabled the person to continue his work as a school teacher throughout the episode.

Summary

The problem-based approach enables clinical management to be targeted to specific problems that are highly relevant to people's everyday functioning. The impairments, disabilities and handicaps that result from major mental disorders are addressed in a comprehensive way that integrates self-help, informal problem solving and multidisciplinary professional strategies. Problems of recent onset as well as long-standing difficulties can all be addressed within this framework. It may appear that such an assessment is very time consuming. For complex cases this indeed may be true, but most straightforward cases can be assessed in 30–40 minutes. It also depends of course whether, as a therapist, one is used to thinking about short-term symptom reduction or longer-term factors such as prevention of problem recurrence and enhancement of each individual's quality of life. The integrated care approach places and appropriate emphasis on accurate diagnosis as a crucial first step which provides a clear direction for biomedical interventions. However we then move on to the detailed assessment strategies that have been outlined, and the distressed person is helped to live as full a life as possible.

It is evident that this problem analysis is targeted to an individual person. It should be noted that the integrated mental health service always attempts to involve at least one informal carer in addition to the index person. These people are assessed in a similar manner, although this assessment may be abbreviated in the manner described in Chapter 7 (pp. 188–223). Additional assessments of the manner in which the people in the care network resolve their problems and achieve their goals as a group are included in this carer assessment. However, the basis of all clinical management is the effort to assist all those who suffer as a result of a mental disorder to restore their expected levels of community functioning as quickly as possible, and to experience minimal social handicaps, regardless of the severity or persistence of the impairment that results from the disorder. The assessment approaches that we have outlined here provide one method of ensuring that the efforts of patients, carers, family practitioner teams, and mental health specialists are fully integrated into an efficient team to achieve these aims.

References

Barlow D.H., Hayes S.C. & Nelson R.O. (1984) *The scientist practitioner.* Pergamon, Oxford.
Brown G.W. & Harris T. (1978) *Social origins of depression: a study of psychiatric disorder in women.* Tavistock, London.
Kanfer F.H. & Saslow G. (1965) Behavioral analysis: an alternative to diagnostic classification. *Archives of General Psychiatry,* **12**, 529–538.
Leff J.P. & Vaughn C.E. (1985) *Expressed emotion in families.* Guilford Press, New York.
Nuechterlein K.H. (1990) Methodological considerations in the search for indicators of vulnerability to severe psychopathology. In J.W. Rorbaugh, R. Johnson, & R. Parasuraman (Eds.) *Event-related potentials of the brain.* Oxford University Press, Oxford.
Shapiro M.B. (1961) A method of measuring psychological changes specific to the individual psychiatric patient. *British Journal of Medical Psychology,* **34**, 151–155.

6

Crisis intervention and intensive care for acute episodes: creating an asylum at home

Despite our best efforts to intervene in the earliest stages of major mental disorders, thereby averting social disability and crises, some people inevitably fail to respond to these early intervention strategies, or present to their family doctors at a later stage in their disorder. Such cases were managed by an *intensive care program*. For the past 100 years the provision of intensive treatment for the mentally disordered has been almost exclusively hospital-based. The focus of early intervention was as much a social function as it is today. The community was considered to be relieved of a potentially dangerous member, who was incarcerated, and provided with basic care. It was considered that such institutions provided an asylum from the stresses of life in the community, but in reality the quality of life in such places was almost identical to that provided in prisons, where no such claims for humanistic benefits were made (Goffman, 1961). During the 1960s with the advent of effective psychosocial and drug treatment strategies, the custodial role of the hospital became less prominent as supportive care gave way to active treatment, and higher rates of admissions and discharges limited the potential to view the hospital as a therapeutic community. The role of mental hospitals as a vehicle for state control of its less well-endowed and dissenting citizens was highlighted by humanists around the globe, with notable contributions from R.D. Laing, Thomas Szasz, Alexander Solzhenitsyn and Franco Basaglia (see Mosher & Burti, 1989). While these crusading figures tended to dramatise rare cases of abuse, they highlighted the excessive zeal of many psychiatrists to enhance their status within medical circles by employing a biomedical model of illness and cure to all persons suffering from mental disorders, and to marginalise the social and

136

environmental factors that contribute to comprehensive models of clinical management (Clare, 1976).

It was not our intent to lead a crusade against hospital care, merely to develop services that met the needs of people suffering the effects of mental disorders who were residing in our community in the most effective and efficient way. It was abundantly clear that a very small proportion of such persons made use of hospital services, and that even those few spent relatively little time in the hospital and most of their time with their friends and families. Yet the hospital service was clearly the focus of most of the therapeutic effort, and consequently absorbed almost all of the budget allocated to the service. Such a disproportionate allocation of resources begged the question of what specific benefits are most effective and efficiently provided by an acute hospital unit.

Hospital admission: the benefits and costs

Before hospital services for the mentally disordered can be replaced it is essential that their benefits are clearly understood and that the replacement services provide identical resources. It is commonly suggested that hospital care is the most effective strategy for the clinical management of suicidal, homicidal and disorganised behaviour associated with schizophrenic and major affective disorders. However, there are no studies to validate these claims. A closer analysis of the specific role the hospital plays in the management of serious behavioural disturbance suggests that the main benefits derive from custodial care and observation of persons, coupled with doses of drugs and ECT that may provoke serious side effects that require frequent medical consultation and nursing supervision. It is clear that these conditions for adequate care are seldom found in peoples' homes, particularly where the individuals concerned are single, live alone, or with friends or relatives who are unable or unwilling to assist in a major way.

A further benefit of hospital care is the ability to monitor neuro-endocrine investigations that require multiple sampling of body fluids at precise times throughout 24-hour periods.

Advocates for expanding hospital-based services consider that another major benefit of hospital care is the asylum provided from the stresses of the non-hospital environment. While it could be argued that the old style mental hospitals provided some semblance of a low stress environment for those people who were encouraged to view them as a home away from home, there is little evidence that the modern acute mental hospital provides effective respite for those that enter its portals. It is extremely difficult to maintain a low stress ambience in a household that contains merely one disturbed person. The expectation that a small staff of well-trained professionals can maintain a similar minimal stress environment when supporting 15 to 20 acutely disturbed people under one roof is highly unrealistic, although it is surprising how effective so many ward regimens are at minimizing serious disturbance when the task is viewed in such straightforward terms.

It can be concluded that the chief benefit of modern psychiatric hospital care is the provision of 24-hour nursing care that enables grossly disturbed behaviour to be safely contained and tolerated, while conducting specialised assessments of that behaviour, monitoring the effects of drugs and other treatment interventions, and conducting specialised neuro-endocrine tests.

Although these benefits are circumscribed, they are far from minimal, and should not be discounted when planning community services. However, they are not achieved without some notable disadvantages. The major disadvantages of treating mental disorders in hospital settings are:

1 Removal of people from their natural habitats and social roles poses added stresses associated with adapting to a strange and often threatening environment. That may cancel out the benefits of escaping from a stressful social network.
2 Highly structured ward environments that contribute substantially to stress management have the disadvantage of encouraging rapid institutionalism.
3 Skills, including coping strategies, that are learned in the hospital are unlikely to generalise to the natural habitat, unless special strategies are employed to promote this transfer of skills.
4 Relief of the burden on informal carers in the social network is often short-lived. Concern for the person's welfare in the disturbed hospital environment, guilt about their role in the admission process, lack of involvement in the person's continued care, taking on the roles that were performed adequately by the person, even

when they were disabled, worry about the person's return home and re-entry into the social network, all serve to reduce the initial relief experienced at the point of hospital admission.

5 The escalating cost of providing accommodation and basic care in a hospital setting progressively reduces the number of people able to benefit from this form of intensive clinical management and leads to rationing on the basis of social rather than medical needs.

Many of these disadvantages apply equally to community-based alternatives to inpatient services where disturbed people are segregated into special programs. In addition, all these disadvantages can be greatly reduced by minimising the time spent in the hospital setting and reducing the boundaries between the hospital and home settings, so that there is freedom of movement and access of all significant persons between these settings. Examples of such integration between inpatient units and community settings are rare despite open-door policies and the abolition of restricted visiting hours. This summary of the benefits of hospital care for acute episodes of mental disorders concludes that the role of the hospital is vital for a comprehensive mental health service, but is relatively more circumscribed than that provided by most current services.

What is needed to replace the mental hospital?

Any alternative to hospital-based intensive care must provide all those services provided by the hospital setting. This includes 24-hour supervision, by adequately skilled persons, easy accessibility to opportunities to preserve and enhance social role functioning, including work activities, the ready availability of specialised assessments from physicians, both psychiatrists and neuro-endocrinologists, psychologists, social workers, etc. The absence of any one of these components will reduce the effectiveness of the service and render it liable to justified criticism that it is inferior to the hospital.

From the clinician's standpoint, there seems little to be gained by changing the locus of treatment of people with mental disorders, unless there is evidence that this change enhances the quality of that treatment and facilitates recovery. From the tax-paying members of the community it may be of secondary concern that an equally effective service can be provided at a lower cost. There is considerable evidence that community-based alternatives to hospitals can provided intensive care for the mentally disordered that is equally effective. There is less evidence that this can be achieved with any substantial cost savings to the community, particularly where the alternative involves the provision of board and lodgings outside the person's home. Four studies of successful intensive care programs will be described briefly to illustrate the benefits and costs of such approaches.

Training in community living program: Dane County, Wisconsin

The intensive care aspects of this program which is the leading example of a community-based service (see Chapter 2, pp. 47–49 for an overview) were developed in the early 1970s by Drs Leonard Stein and Mary Ann Test. A hospital ward was closed and its staff redeployed in the community. In a controlled study, people presenting with psychiatric crises and needing intensive care were randomly assigned to either routine hospital services or to community-based alternatives. The Training in Community Living program assigned a case manager to each person. The case manager returned home with the disturbed individual and provided them with the support to continue their daily activities in the community. Psychiatric and psychological consultation was provided from a team based in a mental health centre, and extensive assistance was provided with sheltered housing and other social needs. Initially, a deliberate policy of removing people from family households was employed, on the theoretical basis that disturbed family relationships were a common feature associated with acute episodes of mental disorders. Thus, considerable efforts were needed to secure alternative housing. Mental health personnel were available throughout the 24 hours and 7 days per week. The services provided were all directed towards improving the social and community living skills of participants, even when they were acutely disturbed by delusional or mood disorders. The services were provided in an assertive manner, ensuring that people did not dropout, and maximised their participation in a full range of work and leisure opportunities in the community. The principles of this program are summarised in Table

Table 6.1. *Conceptual model of the Training in Community Living program. TCL considered these components as essential requirements for a successful community-based mental health program*

Material resources, such as food, shelter, clothing, and general medical care

Coping skills to meet the demands of community life. These include use of public transportation, preparing nutritious meals, budgeting money. Training should take place *in situ*, where the skills are needed and used

Motivation to persevere and remain involved in life, particularly when faced with overwhelming stress. Training in real-life problem resolution and personal support by therapists

Freedom from pathologically dependent relationships that inhibit personal growth, reinforce maladaptive behaviour, and generate panic when their loss is threatened. This includes institutional and family care. Efforts to encourage growth towards greater autonomy are emphasised

Support and education of all community members who are involved with patients. This includes family, police, landlords, and various community agencies

A support system that *assertively* helps the patient with the previous five requirements with proactive outreach and other efforts to ensure that the patient receives the help he or she requires at the time it is required

---

6.1. A two-month training period was provided before each professional began work on the program.

The results of this well-controlled study indicated that such an approach was not only feasible, but that over a 14-month period it resulted in superior symptom management, social role functioning, including work activity, and minimal utilisation of hospital resources (Stein & Test, 1980). Furthermore, there was no evidence that family members or other community resources experienced any extra burden as a consequence of this approach (Test & Stein, 1980). However, the extensive care provided in the community did not allow for any reduction in overall costs compared with the hospital service. Although a benefit–cost analysis suggested that there was greater efficiency achieved by providing a service in this manner (Weisbrod et al, 1980).

It is important to note that this approach provided continued treatment for people after their acute crises had been controlled. For many severely disabled people this amounted to personalised day treatment, and resulted in extremely close ties developing with case managers. A major problem arose when the project attempted to return participants to standard community mental health care. A rapid loss of benefits was noted. This suggests that such a model requires continuity of supportive treatment, and that factors such as changes in case managers may adversely affect the maintenance of progress previously achieved. It is apparent that the same sort of dependence fostered by hospitals and other institutions can arise in the community, and that further research is needed to establish the optimal blend of skills training and support for those severely disabled by mental disorders.

The Montreal Project

Fred Fenton and his colleagues in Montreal (1981) conducted a very similar project at around the same time that the TCL program was developing. The project was remarkably similar, although suicidal patients were excluded, in addition to the substance abuse problems and organic brain disorders excluded in the Wisconsin study. A sample of 162 people needing intensive crisis management were randomly assigned to either routine hospital care or the Home Treatment program. This program was less intensive than TCL, with less emphasis on living skills training and more on crisis family interventions of the kind pioneered by Don Langsley in Denver (Langsley et al, 1971), and Denis Scott at Napsbury Hospital in England (Scott, 1974). People assigned to home-based care spent two-thirds less time in hospital than those routinely-treated. This led to considerable cost savings for this approach. No differences were observed in the efficiency of symptom relief, burden on carers, or overall social functioning. However, it was noted that most people receiving home-based care were able to continue to carry out at least some of their responsibilities at work and at home even while in considerable distress. This spared family members from taking on the additional responsibilities that result when a person is admitted to hospital.

The Sydney Project

The Sydney Project (Hoult, 1986) resembled the Montreal approach. The focus was on crisis intervention, with less emphasis on long-term skill training. The results of a random controlled trial of 120 cases of people with florid episodes of functional psychoses

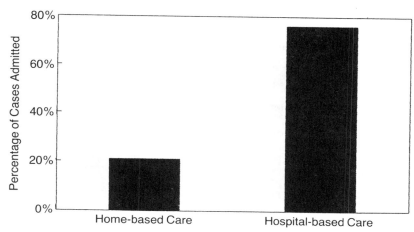

Figure 6.1. Hospital admissions during one-year of follow-up after home-based and hospital-based emergency care. (From Stein & Test, 1980; Hoult et al, 1981.)

were very similar, with substantial cost savings and greater patient and carer satisfaction for the home-based service.

A recent attempt to replicate these controlled research projects at the Maudsley Hospital, London, has made greater use of brief periods of hospital care than the earlier studies, and provides less out of hours treatment. Preliminary results suggest that the advantages of the home-based approach are broadly similar to those found in the previous work (Muijen et al, 1992).

It may be concluded that around 80% of crisis admissions to mental hospitals can be averted where home-based intensive treatment can be provided, preferably on a 24-hour basis. Clinical and social recovery are achieved with similar efficiency to that achieved in hospital settings, role functioning is preserved at least to some extent, and carer burden is not increased (Figures 6.1 and 6.2).

Only one of the research studies has adequately addressed the needs for training in living skills and stress management that is considered vital to improving the quality of life of people suffering mental disorders and to reducing the risk of further acute episodes. It is considered crucial that the intensive care program is an integral part of a comprehensive mental health service, and that continuity of active interventions are ensured until it appears certain that long-term mental health can be assured after transfer back to primary

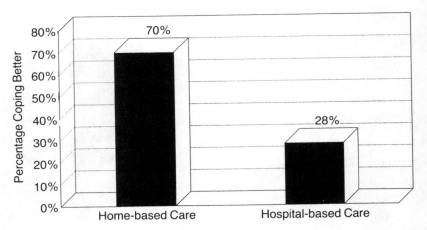

Figure 6.2. Percentage of carers reporting that they coped better with patients' problems during one-year of follow-up after home-based and hospital-based emergency care. (From Hoult, 1986.)

care resources. In some cases this treatment program may need to extend indefinitely (Test et al, 1985).

The integrated approach to home-based intensive care

In the integrated care model two major modifications have been made to the intensive home-based care programs outlined above: (1) a greater focus on training carers in clinical management skills, including stress management approaches; and (2) the initiation of intensive intervention long before people were considered in need of hospital admission. In most other respects the approach resembles those controlled demonstrations that have repeatedly shown that the majority of people admitted to mental institutions could be treated effectively and efficiently in the comfort of their own home environments.

The components of home-based intensive care

The home-based intensive care program consists of the following components:

1 Referral consultation and family practitioner screening.
2 Patient assessment.
3 Carer assessment.
4 Initial intervention contract.
5 Training the patient and carer in crisis stress management.
6 Monitoring and reviewing progress in a systematic way.
7 Training in specific strategies for specific problem behaviours.

Once the most florid aspects of the crisis have been resolved efforts then focus on preventing recurrent episodes with continued psycho-social rehabilitation to overcome residual disability. These aspects are described in subsequent chapters.

It is worth noting that these components are identical to those associated with intensive care in hospital. However, we have attempted to specify these procedures in a clear and systematised manner, so that each member of the service fully comprehends the nature of the particular tasks are requested to perform. We note that the trend towards defining the process and goals of mental health nursing encompasses these aims, and applaud this move. However, we venture to suggest that such structure needs to include all members of the multidisciplinary team (including the family practitioners), so that collaboration is optimal and misunderstanding minimal.

Referral consultation and screening by the family practitioner

Following a screening assessment, consultation concerning the need for intensive care is initiated at the request of a person's family practitioner, who, in some cases may have been alerted to the crisis by another community agency, such as a hospital emergency service, local social services, or police. In some cases this screening is a formality and without delay the family practitioner immediately calls in the mental health specialists. However, frequently the family practitioner may decide to assess the person before deciding whether expert assistance is indicated. This is most common where someone is currently receiving treatment from the primary care professionals, who feel confident that they would be able to continue to provide effective clinical management.

An example was a 37-year-old woman in the early stages of her second pregnancy, who was referred directly to the mental health service by a consultant obstetrician for management of her depressive symptoms, including thoughts of suicide. Her family doctor knew her well, was providing her antenatal care, and knew that her symptoms and self-destructive thoughts had been a constant feature since early adulthood. This had led to occasional episodes of excessive drinking. He had succeeded in counselling her to remain abstinent throughout this pregnancy, and had been seeing her weekly during the first trimester, for psychological support when she had felt unwell with unremitting nausea. He felt that a specialist mental health assessment would not help at this stage, and might prove particularly upsetting. A brief discussion with the psychiatrist affirmed this plan, with the understanding that continued informal consultation with the mental health service would be provided. The psychiatrist suggested that the family doctor assessed the woman's depressive symptoms on each visit, particularly her sleep and appetite (after the nausea wore off), as well as feelings of hopelessness and self-destruction. A note of the specific mental status questions used to assess these symptoms in a standardised manner was made in her antenatal file so that he could refer to this each time he met the patient. As predicted by the family doctor, the mood disturbance remained stable, improving somewhat during the later stages of pregnancy. Excellent additional support from the community midwife and health visitor enabled the family practice team to deal with the childbirth and post-natal period without exacerbation of emotional symptoms. Brief consultation with a mental health therapist was provided over coffee on two additional occasions and strategies that aimed to enhance this woman's low self-esteem were suggested to the health visitor. Application of these strategies appeared to assist in the successful management of this case.

In every case where an urgent request for mental health consultation is made, it is expected that the family practitioner has either already completed his own assessment of the case, or is planning a joint assessment with the mental health professional on duty at the practice. Apart from screening the mental status of the patient to decide whether a request for mental health assessment is indicated, the family practitioner is requested to conduct an assessment of those general medical aspects of the case that might be relevant to the differential diagnosis and clinical management. Aspects of medical history are reviewed and relevant systems examined. Where any abnormality is suspected, appropriate biomedical screening is carried out. Examples include blood counts for anaemia, urine and blood sugar for diabetes, X-rays and EEGs for headaches, or neurological signs. We believe that the family practitioner is the most appropriate expert to take responsibility for screening underlying medical conditions, with consultation from team psychiatrists, as well as from other medical specialists.

This specific role of the family practitioner in the assessment of a crisis presentation ensures that the doctor is an integral member of the therapeutic team throughout any period of intensive care, and does not withdraw from the clinical process after it has been decided that extensive specialised mental health resources are needed.

We mentioned previously that a mental health therapist is available in each practice throughout all clinic hours. A radiopager and mobile telephone enable rapid contact at all other times throughout a 24-hour period, including weekends. We aim for a maximum of 10 minutes delay contacting the person requesting consultation, and 20 minutes delay in beginning a specialised assessment of each case. With few exceptions, these goals were readily met. Weekday assessments are conducted by staff assigned to the patient's own primary care team. However, consultation after hours and at weekends are covered by designated staff, who cover several primary care teams. These rosters include all members of the mental health service, not merely the nursing therapists, with the psychiatrists providing much of the night consultation work. This often amounts to telephone discussion with a family practitioner, with night visits proving rare, at least after 8 p.m. The family practitioners reported that they felt more confident in their own ability to manage overnight crises, knowing that they could readily call for help, and that the case would receive immediate attention the next morning.

Record keeping associated with requests for consultation is made as efficient as possible with the family practitioner completing the Presenting Problems, Reasons for Referral and Current Management sections of the Community Health Record card (see Appendix 1). The remainder of the record is completed by the mental health therapist. The record is kept in the patients' primary care record file at all times so that all members of the primary care team have ready access to it whenever they are deputising for the doctor and mental health therapist who made the initial assessment.

Initial assessment

The main goals of the crisis assessment are to:

1 Establish rapport with the patient.
2 Target the key problems.
3 Define the role that a mental disorder may be playing in the origin and maintenance of these problems.

Establishing rapport

The importance of establishing excellent rapport with the distressed person cannot be overemphasised. So often people perceive their mental health crisis as one in which they are the victims of life circumstances, manipulated by people in their immediate social network, who more often than not will have instigated the consultation. The ability of the therapist to persuade the patient that he or she is acting first and foremost in the interests of preserving or maintaining their quality of life is crucial to reducing the fear associated with an unwanted intrusion into the distressed person's personal affairs. We advocate that the therapist immediately greets the patient upon entering their home, and tells other family members and friends that he intends to assess the patient before assessing the family members. The presence of the family doctor in the initial interview may assist in reducing tension, particularly if he or she is well known to the patient. Certainly where the risk of violence is suspected it is crucial that another person accompanies the therapist, doors are left ajar, and, if the risk appears high, that police are in close attendance.

The therapist should introduce himself by briefly explaining the reason for his assessment, what he aims to achieve, and how long he expects to take. For example:

> Jill, I am a therapist working in Doctor Smith's practice, and he has asked me to help him find some ways of helping you with the problems that seem to be upsetting you at the moment. I would like to ask you a few questions about those problems so that I can get a better idea about them. That will probably take about half an hour. I would like

Dr. Smith to stay with us because he knows you better than me and may be able to help. Is that OK for you?

It is important to recognise that non-verbal aspects of communication may have a profound impact upon rapport. We advise therapists wherever possible to conduct interviews in the comfort of the living room, choosing to sit a comfortable distance from the patient on chairs of similar heights, arranged in such a manner that eye contact is easily maintained. Distractions from music and television should be minimised, by polite requests to patient and family. At times, if the person is bedridden he/she may be asked to get up, or at least to sit comfortably. A chair may be requested so that the therapist is able to sit next to the bed. Conducting interviews while standing over a supine patient may be perceived as threatening and sitting on a person's bed may be perceived as too intimate.

The same principles that apply to good interviewing in outpatient and hospital settings are applicable in the home. However, it is crucial to realise that you are a guest of the household and that appropriate social customs and manners should be closely adhered to. Much can be learned about the practical aspects of home assessment from other members of the primary care team, who may have considerable experience of handling medical crises at home. They may provide invaluable guidance about the cultural values of the household, which in addition to ethnic issues, may include religious practices, attitudes to authority, and a variety of customs that may be crucial to the context of your visit. Failure to take account of these issues may imperil your venture.

Targeting the key problems

A major part of the crisis assessment entails defining the exact nature of the patient's presenting problems. It is important to note that these are the *patient's* problems, not those of the family or neighbours, who may have experienced problems of their own as a consequence of the patient's behaviour. Of course in many cases the patient's behaviour may be a response to the behaviour of those around him, and crises are usually compounded by vicious circles of this nature.

We have discussed the problem-oriented assessment process in Chapter 5. The same assessment methods are used when dealing with people in crisis situations, though the focus tends to be on

immediate difficulties and their antecedents. The targeting of problems involves inviting the patient to describe exactly what he or she
has experienced as the major impairments leading to his or her
current predicament. These may be symptoms, such as 'I have a
feeling of overwhelming fear that I'm about to die' or 'I hear the
neighbours saying that I'm an IRA bomber through my bedroom
wall', or 'I just have no energy at all'. Alternatively, they may be
responses associated with the symptoms, such as 'I cannot concentrate on what I'm doing; I keep forgetting things all the time', or 'I
am upset that my husband wants sex and I have no desire at all'.

Further assessment aims to clarify the precise nature of the
experiences in terms of frequency, intensity and modifying or coping
factors. This questioning leads to a redefinition of the problem in a
more specific way. For example, the problem of 'not sleeping at all'
may become . . .

> 'Sleeping between 2 and 3 hours at night between the hours of 2
>   and 5 a.m. without sleeping tablets; and 1 hour during the
>   evening when watching television'
> 'Started 12 days ago after my wife told me she is having an affair'
> 'Made better by sleeping in the spare room, and taking sleeping
>   tablets prescribed by my doctor – 4–5 hours per night – but
>   tablet effects less beneficial in past 3 days'
> 'Worse if I have a discussion with my wife about her affair; if I
>   drink more than 5 half-pint mugs of coffee'
> 'Better if I go to bed around midnight'
> 'I would be able to perform better at my work and be less irritable
>   with my wife if I could get a good night's sleep, but she would be
>   less concerned about me and might leave me'

No more than two problems are targeted in this way at the initial
assessment. These are chosen in terms of the disability that appears
to stem from them and are not always symptoms that are key to the
diagnosis of a mental disorder. For example, problems with sleep
tend to have a major impact, not merely on the every day functioning
of patients, but frequently lead to disturbance for all household
members, yet they are seldom specific features of any mental
disorder and occur in all forms of stress related circumstances.
Severely reduced appetite of similarly recent onset, on the other
hand, has much greater diagnostic specificity, yet can be present for
some days or weeks before it is likely to affect a person's everyday

functioning. Therefore, in choosing a target problem for initial intervention a therapist would be more likely to prioritise a severe sleep problem. However, that does not mean that a problem with major long-term consequences, such as reduced appetite, would not be the target of intervention strategies from the onset of intensive treatment.

A key aspect of this problem-oriented crisis assessment involves assessment of the way in which the patient attempts to cope with the problems. Even in situations of major crisis, people employ a whole range of coping strategies which therapists can build on. All self-help efforts to ameliorate and compensate for the problem are noted, including those that appear to have negative consequences, and may indeed be adding to long-term disability and handicap. Special note is made of problem-solving efforts made in collaboration with carers and other resources in the community. It is surprising how often people and their carers employ all the strategies recommended in nursing and psychology manuals for their particular disorders. Their lack of success in the application of these strategies appears to be less often due to their lack of resourcefulness, than due to their failure to persist with strategies that are not immediately rewarding, or to employ them in the systematic manner used in effective therapeutic applications. A survey of 40 people with persisting auditory hallucinations (Falloon & Talbot, 1981) revealed the following range of coping strategies:

Engaged in leisure activity   73%
Change of posture (e.g. sit, lie, stand, walk)   63%
Initiated interpersonal contact   48%
Engaged in work activity   28%
Took extra dose of prescribed medication   28%
Considered suicidal activity   28%
Took non-prescribed drugs (alcohol, analgesics, illicit
    drugs)   25%
Social withdrawal   5%

Clearly some of these tactics are more effective than others, but it is unwise to make such a judgement prior to detailed enquiry about the precise manner in which the strategy is employed, and the advantages and disadvantages that the person perceives when he or she applies the strategy in any specific context. Well-validated strategies, such as exposure to feared objects in the treatment of phobias, often appear inappropriate and paradoxical when first suggested. Thus, the benefits of all coping strategies should be balanced with their detrimental effects and costs to the person using them.

A further benefit from examining the manner in which a person copes with impairments is that among the various strategies is often one or more that has been validated as a helpful therapeutic strategy. This approach may be one that is seldom employed. Nevertheless it indicates to the therapist that the person already has the strategy in his or her repertoire and that therapy may merely need to promote the more frequent and consistent use of the strategy, rather than to train the person in the rudiments of the method. The impaired person is thus seen as a creative, effective individual, who is continually attempting to enhance his or her coping abilities, rather than a passive recipient of the treatment provided only through the expertise of the omnipotent therapist. This partnership between therapist and patient is seen as a key component of all aspects of the integrated therapy approach outlined in this book.

Defining the association between the mental disorder and key problems

The precise association between suspected mental disorders and key problems needs to be clearly delineated. Most members of the community, including professionals providing primary care services, tend to equate disturbed or bizarre behaviour with serious mental disorder. However, most people displaying such behaviour disturbance are not formally mentally disordered. They are more often displaying ineffective coping strategies in response to overwhelming life problems. A crucial role that the specialist mental health professional must play in the community is to help clarify those cases of behaviour disturbance that are associated with mental disorders, and those that are not. In order to carry out this task, it is crucial that all members of the mental health service are trained to make reliable diagnostic assessments, and share common criteria for determining whether or not someone is suffering from a mental disorder. The ability to present a consistent response to community agencies when they request assistance with the management of disturbed citizens is considered one of the most important aspects of our approach. The value of the biopsychosocial model of mental disorders is limited to people who show the characteristic features of mental disorders, and may actually harm others to whom it is applied. For example, a person responding to a bereavement may show some features similar to a depressive disorder, or a person under excessive work stress may exhibit features found in generalised anxiety disorders, or an eccentric, reclusive person features similar to chronic schizophrenia. None of these people is likely to benefit from being treated in the same manner as those experiencing mental disorders. In particular, the benefits of drug treatments and other medical procedures are unlikely to produce the benefits associated with their application when employed to alter the pathophysiological states associated with mental disorders. Psychosocial strategies may of course assist in overcoming disability and handicaps, and may possibly reduce any risks of mental or physical ill health, particularly in those people deemed vulnerable by virtue of specific genetic, clinical background, or psychosocial factors.

On the other hand, people with mental disorders who appear to be coping effectively with their adverse life problems, are often deprived of the benefits of mental health expertise because primary caregivers fail to recognise mental disorders in the absence of gross social disturbance.

We believe that a successful community-based service must adhere to the highest standards of psychiatric assessment present in excellent hospitals. Any diminution in the ability to define mental disorders will lead to the service deploying more resources attempting to treat people experiencing primary psychosocial disturbance with inappropriate and ineffective methods, and reduce the ability to provide effective clinical management of those people disabled by mental disorders, who respond in a predictable way to the state-of-the-art treatment methods outlined in Chapter 3.

Once the key problems of the disturbed person have been clarified, a standardised mental health history is completed. This provides a screening of potential risk factors for mental disorders, such as the history of previous episodes and response to treatment, family history, stress and vulnerability factors, including poor premorbid adjustment, life events, social stressors, and substance abuse.

The patient assessment is completed with a diagnostic assessment using the Present State Examination interview (Wing et al, 1974). The entire PSE may be completed, or, where the therapist is confident that the presentation is more specific, ratings derived from part of the interview may be completed. The section concerning depressive symptoms may be completed and rated on the Hamilton Rating Scale for Depression. Similar rating scales have been derived for manic episodes, anxiety disorders and schizophrenia, that combine the standardised interview strategies of the PSE with standard ratings of severity, from which diagnostic classifications can be easily determined. Because the diagnostic classification system developed for the PSE is designed for computer analysis, we chose to employ the American Psychiatric Association's diagnostic system, DSM-III. This provides mental health specialists from all disciplines with a series of checklists that enable symptoms and historical information to be translated into the criteria for psychiatric syndromes in a highly consistent fashion. Every therapist entering the service is trained to the rigorous standards established for agreement between raters in major research studies (reliability between their ratings and that of an expert exceeding 0.80 on item agreement) before conducting crisis assessments. Continuing case presentations and follow-up workshops ensure that high levels of competence are maintained.

The completion of both problem analysis and diagnostic assessment then presents the therapist with the problem of reconciling the association between the two. The impairment of a mental disorder may be the major factor underlying the disabling problems the patient experiences, such as the case where intense preoccupation with unpleasant thoughts hinders concentration and memory functions, and handicap the person in his or her roles at work. Treatment of the symptom of excessive worrying thoughts would be likely to resolve the cognitive deficiencies that make work activity difficult. However, such direct associations between symptoms and problems are not universal, and some problems may be independent of the symptoms. For example, a person suffering identical worrying thoughts, who considers his or her key problem to be difficulty establishing convivial relationships in the workplace may lack an effective repertoire of social skills. This is unlikely to be alleviated merely by resolution of his or her worrying. Formulating the disorder in clear-cut terms is seldom possible after the initial interview with the person in crisis. However, it is essential that the therapist is able to establish some priorities for immediate intervention, whilst leaving the patient in no doubt that he or she will receive comprehensive assistance with all his or her perceived

difficulties in a holistic manner. A simple explanation of the therapist's preliminary formulation may prove very reassuring to the
disturbed person at this stage, particularly if the therapist seeks the
patient's view on the plausibility of this formulation. An example of
this may be:

> You seem to me to be suffering from a moderately severe depressive
> disorder, similar to the one you had 18 months ago. Possibly the upset
> you have had at work may have brought this on at this time, although
> it seems to me that you are gradually getting depressed over the past
> few months, while your sleep has been poor. I would like to help you
> overcome some of your worrying first and then see if we can see if you
> can find some ways to cope with your difficulties at work. Does that
> sound reasonable to you?

It may not be possible to conduct a detailed assessment of this
kind in one sitting with severely distressed individuals. However, the
therapist is able to spend several hours with people, during which
brief assessment discussions can be interspersed with periods when
they are encouraged to participate in everyday activities appropriate
to their current levels of functioning. This helps reduce the tension of
the interview process, while contributing to the therapist's understanding of the disorder and its impact on functioning. Such an
approach merely replicates good nursing practice in hospital settings. It has the major advantage of observing the person in natural
surroundings where behavioural patterns are less likely to be distorted. The daily fluctuations of impairments and the manner in
which patients' and carers' efforts to cope contribute to recovery,
maintenance or worsening of the disorder can be observed.

Crisis assessment of carers and the care network

The patient's key informal carers are interviewed using the semi-
structured Family Member Interview (Falloon et al, 1988). In
addition to background information about their own health status,
including their own vulnerability to stress-related health problems,
their understanding of the patient's suspected disorder, ability to
cope with the main behaviour problems, and their subjective and
objective burdens associated with caring are assessed. The interview
is conducted in privacy and permits carers to clearly express their

concerns and personal distress. This method is based upon the well-known research-based Camberwell Family Interview approach (Vaughn & Leff, 1976). However, ratings of emotional responses are not made routinely, and the Expressed Emotion index is not employed. Rather, the strengths and weaknesses of the carer are assessed in terms of coping effectively with the current crisis and the need for specific professional assistance.

In the initial assessment of those caring for distressed people it is essential to decide whether or not the person can be managed most effectively at home. To help us to make that decision we address the following points:

1 Can informal care provide effective support for that person in terms of basic requirements of lodgings, food, hygiene, etc?
2 Can informal care provide assistance in monitoring the person's disturbed behaviour, including potentially dangerous behaviour?
3 To what extent may the living environment contribute to alleviation of the disorder?
4 To what extent may the living environment contribute to the maintenance or worsening of the disorder?
5 To what extent would removal of the person from the home environment alleviate the disorder?
6 To what extent would removal of the person from the home environment exacerbate the disorder, or contribute to long-term disability or handicap?
7 How would removal of the person from the home environment benefit/handicap informal carers?

These questions can be summarised in terms of seeking the optimal biopsychosocial environment in which to alleviate the distress associated with the present crisis, not only for the people suffering from mental disorders, but also for their informal carers. However, it is important to note that the interests of the distressed sufferer should not be supplanted by the interests of the distressed carer. Nor should convenience to the professional services be a primary consideration in formulating intervention strategies.

A simple decision tree that outlines the reasons for choosing a hospital setting for clinical management of a crisis is provided in *Figure 6.3*. It should be noted that under present UK mental health legislation (Mental Health Act, 1983) it is not possible to provide

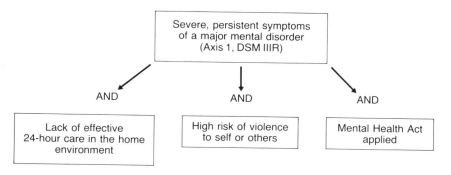

NOTE: Intensive treatment plan continues regardless of where person is currently residing (e.g. home, hospital, prison)

Figure 6.3. Criteria for admission to a psychiatric inpatient unit.

home-based management of anyone considered mentally disordered and likely to behave in a manner that could endanger his or her own life or that of others. While it is difficult to assess dangerousness, there is little evidence that admission to a mental hospital is prophylactic. Such admissions merely transfer the risk to another setting, where fellow patients become potential victims, and surveillance by staff may prove even more difficult than in the home setting. Nevertheless, violence and death in mental hospital settings appear to engender less protest from the community than that in the home setting. Such attitudes perpetuate the discrimination against the mentally disordered, who are seldom encouraged to press charges against fellow sufferers who assault them on the wards, or complain to hospital authorities when the suicide of an associate adds to their distress. Clearly where mental disorders contribute directly to dangerous behaviour citizens need 24-hour care and treatment in an environment that preserves the safety of themselves and their fellow citizens. It should not be assumed that this can only be achieved in a hospital ward. Such decisions should involve the family and wherever possible, the patient. Furthermore, decisions should be made with full understanding of the advantages and disadvantages of management in the variety of settings available. Such problem solving tends to defuse many distressing family crises, and frequently enables the patient to accept a short-term admission to a hospital unit without acrimony and the need to resort to legal action. An example of this was the case of Mr S.

Mr S was a 62-year old man, who had been made redundant from a longstanding job 18 months earlier. He lived with a mildly retarded son, and had three married children in the neighbourhood, who provided everyday support to their household. They were not surprised when he appeared distressed after leaving work. But this distress continued and he gradually experienced deterioration in his sleep and appetite, with increasing feelings of hopelessness. These features engendered increasing family support, but they did not contact their family doctor until Mr S threatened suicide. Within 20 minutes of their contact with the doctor the patient had been assessed by a mental health therapist, who considered that the patient was a serious suicide risk. A family meeting was convened within an hour. Mr S was initially adamant that he did not want to go to a hospital. The following alternatives are considered:

    stay at home with constant supervision from mental health service
    stay with a son who runs a pub
    go to the community hospital
    go to a nearby nursing home
    stay at home with constant family supervision only

Each of the options was considered in terms of the main advantages and disadvantages to both patient and carers. It became clear that the house and equipment was in very poor repair and that many of his worries centred on his inability to carry out essential repairs. This contributed to increasing dependence on family support for cooking meals, bathing, laundry, etc. The family agreed to carry out a major overhaul of all household equipment and to redecorate the living room during the course of the next two weeks. Mr S agreed that a brief stay in a psychiatric unit would enable this work to be conducted efficiently. His disabled son would stay at the pub during this time. Within 10 days Mr S had shown substantial improvement and returned home to assist in the household repairs. The family were trained to encourage their father to develop a range of constructive daily activities inside and outside the home, and to avoid carrying out tasks on his behalf without his contributions.

A key concern for carers is the ability to provide 24-hour supervision of a disturbed person. Work and social commitments often make it very difficult for families and friends to sustain such efforts, even when they are keen to do so. Carers who initially express rejection of continuation of their caring role frequently welcome such a role, when they are told that they will receive substantial relief and support for that role from the home-based service. Others will express concern about having a team of professionals taking over their roles. We maintain the policy of not taking over roles that the carers are willing and able to carry out themselves. However, it is essential that informal carers (or professional carers for that matter!) are not expected to perform roles in which they are not competent. These roles must be taken by appropriately qualified professionals. Alternatively, carers may receive training in the skills required and carry out the tasks under the supervision of the professional team. The skills needed will vary according to the nature of each individual's disorder, but three key skills are (1) assessment of target problem behaviours; (2) maintenance of constructive patterns for the patient; and (3) maintaining adherence to drug therapy regimens. It is difficult to assess the carers' competence on the initial visit and it is usually necessary for the therapist to observe these skills during a more extended period, and to carry out any training needed in the real life setting. It should be emphasised again, that at no time do we expect informal carers to care for people unwillingly, and at no stage is any coercion exerted upon unwilling carers. More frequently therapists express their own concern that carers are burdened, and tend to err on the side of offering more assistance than necessary. Carers are encouraged to continue their work and social activities outside the home while staff are in attendance. The availability of secondary carers in the household and social network is assessed, and the support that they may be able to provide is evaluated. Assistance from such sources with practical tasks such as cooking, cleaning or laundry may greatly relieve the primary carers. On occasions social services may provide home care assistants to support families in this way. When patients are admitted to hospital similar efforts are made to involve carers, and to assist in the practical difficulties that may result, both in terms of attendance at hospital and in supporting child care and household functions in the absence of the patient. This is particularly important when the patient is involved in child care and home management. Of course where other adults are living in the household, the service attempts to train them in any skills that they may need to deploy. The assistance of a social worker and occupational therapist with these issues has, for example, enabled fathers to enhance their childrearing and home management skills during periods when their wives have been out of the home. Many of these important issues are not adequately addressed in hospital-based services. As a consequence family tensions are heightened as a result of many hospital admissions that leave many ill-prepared people literally holding the baby!

The initial contract

At the conclusion of the initial crisis assessment, and if it is agreed that the distressed person could be cared for at home, the therapist devises an initial contract that is based upon his or her provisional formulation of the nature of the crisis. A major aim is to minimise clinical, social and carer morbidity with maximum efficiency. This contract needs to include the following elements:

  assessment of target problems/symptoms
  specific strategies to be carried out by the patient
  specific strategies to be carried out by the carer(s)
  specific strategies to be carried out by the mental health team
  procedures for reviewing progress
  procedures for handling emergencies

Although each element of the contract may be quite straightforward, the overall plan may involve several steps. It is, therefore, usually essential to write down procedures for the benefit of all concerned. A copy of the plan is left in a prominent place in the home, as well as in the patient's medical records. It is crucial that the plan is clearly agreed by all important parties, both the patient and carers as well as the mental health professional team. This may not be feasible immediately, but should be accomplished within 24 hours. The presence of any member of the integrated care team who is opposed to the plan may prove sufficient to undermine the entire venture.

The assessment of the one or two specific problems or symptoms considered the major current concern is aided by ensuring that they are clearly defined in everyday language, so that all involved are able to conduct valid ratings of their severity. A specific rating sheet is devised for each problem. This is completed by the patient and/or carers and the professional staff at clearly specified intervals, in order to indicate the progress of each problem. An example of such ratings is provided in Figure 6.4.

These ratings are reviewed daily by the key therapist and upon each visit by other assisting clinicians. Changes in the therapeutic regimen are made contingent upon changes in the target problems.

DATES	ACTIVITY/DURATION	TALK ABOUT WORRYING THOUGHTS 0 – NONE 2 – SLIGHT 4 – MODERATE 6 – MARKED 8 – SEVERE	SLEEP DURATION	MEDICATION TAKEN
a.m.	Housework / Shopping	5 / 2		8am Mellaril 200mg ✓
p.m.	Gardening / Watching TV	3 / 7	3.5 hours	12 midday Mellaril 100mg ✓
Eve.	Eating dinner / Watching TV	6 / 4		8pm Mellaril 200mg ✓
a.m.	Housework	4		8am Mellaril 200mg ✓
p.m.	Going for walk / Going for drive	4 / 5	4 hours	12 midday Mellaril 200mg ✓
Eve.	Listening to music	2		8pm Mellaril 200mg ✓
a.m.	Walking Susan to school / Shopping	1 / 2		8am Mellaril 200mg ✓
p.m.	Cleaning bedroom	6	4 hours	12 midday Mellaril 200mg ✓
Eve.	Preparing dinner / Going for walk	3 / 3		8pm Mellaril 200mg ✓
a.m.	Walking Susan to school / Housework	0 / 4		8am Mellaril 200mg ✓
p.m.	Visiting friends	2	5.5 hours	12 midday Mellaril 200mg ✓
Eve.	Going for drive / Watching TV	2 / 5		8pm Mellaril 200mg ✓
a.m.	Walking Susan to school / Shopping	0 / 2		8am Mellaril 200mg ✓
p.m.	Preparing lunch	2	4 hours	12 midday Mellaril 200mg ✓
Eve.	Housework / Watching TV	4 / 4		9.30 pm Mellaril 200mg ✓
a.m.	Lying in bed	7		8am Mellaril 200mg ✓
p.m.	Therapist session / Playing piano	6 / 3	2 hours.	12 midday Mellaril 200mg ✓
Eve.	Watching TV	6		9.00 pm Mellaril 200mg ✓
a.m.	Walking Susan to school / Sitting in lounge	4 / 8		8am Mellaril 200mg ✓
p.m.	Lying in bed	7	1.5 hours	12 midday Mellaril 200mg ✓
Eve.	Watching TV / Lying in bed	8 / 8		9.00pm Mellaril ✓
a.m.	Shopping / Cooking cake	2 / 3		8am Mellaril 200mg ✓
p.m.	Playing piano	2	4.5 hours	12 midday Mellaril 200mg ✓
Eve.	Watching TV / Preparing dinner	3 / 4		9.00 pm Mellaril 200mg ✓

Figure 6.4. A problem rating chart.

The specific strategies to be carried out by the patient are clearly specified. In addition to positive actions, such as taking prescribed medication at specified times in specified doses, or carrying out specific therapeutic procedures, such as relaxation exercises, or scheduled activities, certain activities may be banned. These may include acting on violent impulses, or self-destructive behaviours. Rather than simply banning such activity, the therapist attempts to get the patient to agree to carry out alternative behaviour at these times. This might include communicating thoughts and feelings about these urges, and contacting specified professionals or agencies. These arrangements are made with the express agreement of the patient as well as any other individuals who are involved. An example of this was a young man who had frequent impulses to jump through a plate glass window. He agreed to tell his mother whenever he felt these impulses strongly, and she agreed to converse with him about everyday things until the impulse diminished. Alternatively, if the impulse failed to go away after 10 minutes of conversation, she would take him for a walk outside. If the impulse persisted the patient agreed to call the therapist immediately.

The precise role of the carer is similarly defined in the initial contract. Particular emphasis is placed on the limits of responsibility and the need to call for professional assistance earlier, rather than later. The usual carer role is similar to that of a nursing assistant in a hospital ward, and care is taken to prevent the carer undertaking duties that should be the prerogative of a skilled nurse. Thus, the carer's duties may include ensuring that the patient receives adequate food, carries out grooming and everyday self-care, takes medication and complies with psychosocial strategies. Of course many carers have acquired exceptional skills of clinical management. Where such skills are evident, and the carer wishes to continue to deploy their expertise, the therapist supports this role, but remains readily available to deputise for the carer at any time. Such support is vital to minimise excessive stress on carers.

The specific strategies that are the responsibility of the mental health service are clearly contracted. These may include a wide range of clinical assessment and therapeutic strategies, provided in sessions that range from one hour per week to 10–12 hours per day, including weekends. Therapeutic intervention is seldom needed after 8 p.m. and an on-call arrangement usually suffices for the occasional assistance needed for individuals who fail to sleep and remain disturbed throughout the night. The family practitioner is usually capable of providing emergency night sedation in such cases, with the assistance of the team psychiatrist for difficult cases. The family doctor remains in charge of the medical management throughout, conducting appropriate diagnostic tests and prescribing all medication, with daily consultation provided by the mental health team. As well as charting target problem severity, records of drug ingestion are kept in the home to ensure that treatment is clearly monitored. Once again these procedures mirror good hospital practice, ensuring that all members of the team, professionals and non-professionals work in an integrated manner. All changes in procedures are clearly noted on the home chart, and are explained to patients, carers, mental health and primary care professionals.

A major concern for patients and their carers is the availability of emergency consultation. The precise details of procedures for seeking such assistance at all times is written on the contract, and rehearsed with the patient and carer to minimise misunderstandings. The family practice remains the first point of call, with mental health professionals available at all times for emergency consultation.

The assistance offered by the therapy team is also clearly agreed between the therapist and the care unit. Times of visits, their duration and the context of therapist involvement is all specified, at least for several days at a time. This enables participants to arrange their lifestyles to accommodate this added intrusion in the most efficient manner. For example, carers and patients may be able to continue at least some aspects of their work or social life outside the household, and therapists are able to continue working with other cases without major disruptions. The crisis management integrates the effective elements of self-help, informal care and professional therapy into a plan that aims to maintain existing levels of functioning of all concerned, and with the expectation that full functioning will be restored as quickly as possible, with minimal additional stress imposed upon any participant. Mutual support and responsibility is made clear in the initial contract. An example of an initial contract is provided in Figure 6.5.

Training patients and carers in crisis stress management

Crisis management remains consistent with the vulnerability and stress model we have employed as a theoretical basis for clinical intervention. It is assumed that a crisis arises when the problems associated with the mental disorder threaten to overwhelm the coping capacity of the individual and his or her care support system.

I, Henry Balder, agree to do the following things:

1. To get out of bed and dress myself before 10.00 a.m. everyday
2. To stay out of my bedroom until 8 p.m.
3. To arrange a schedule of potentially rewarding activities for the next day every evening with assistance from Penny.
4. To tell Penny when I am feeling frustrated and begin to think that life is not worth going on with, even when she is busy.
5. To meet with David for at least two hours everyday from today for the next four days. Times and activities to be planned daily.
6. To take two 75 mg tablets of nortryptiline around 8 p.m. every night, and record any suspected benefits and unwanted effects on checklist every morning.
7. Keep daily records of sleep and activities with help from Penny and David when requested.

I, Penny Balder, agree to do the following:

1. Provide Henry with three light meals daily, to be served at the kitchen table, allowing him to relax and eat slowly.
2. To praise Henry for even his smallest efforts.
3. To supervise his tablet taking each evening.
4. To help him arrange a daily schedule of activities he finds rewarding.
5. To assist in completing ratings.
6. To contact Dr Wyatt and his practice team (including David and Samantha) at anytime of day or night that I am concerned about any aspects of Henry's disorder, or my own coping abilities.

Phone numbers: Dr Wyatt 0280 847 932 daytime
0280 826 434 nights

I, David Jackson, Mental Health Therapist, agree to do the following:

1. To visit Henry and Penny at least once daily for the next four days, for at least two hours.
2. To arrange treatment aimed to increase Henry's time engaged in activities he finds rewarding; and to help him to increase the time he sleeps between 10 p.m. and 8 a.m.
3. To review progress from ratings and discussions everyday and to change plans accordingly.
4. To discuss problems and plans with Dr Wyatt, Samantha James and the mental health team and provide regular reports to them and in Henry's medical record at the practice.

This contract will be reviewed on 23rd March at 4 p.m. It may be terminated before then by any of the parties.

Signed:

H.J. Balder   Penny Balder   D.C. Jackson

Figure 6.5. An intensive care contract.

This may be contingent upon an increase in the severity of impairment as a response to increased biological vulnerability (e.g. hormonal changes), which may be triggered by increased psychosocial stress. Alternatively, an individual who has a persisting level of impairment may show a reduction in coping capacity and may be unable to continue efforts to compensate for the disability that results.

Such 'burnout' may be associated with increases in stress levels, or a reduction in the supportive efforts of carers, who in turn may be incapacitated by stresses in their personal lives. These complex systemic relationships result in a crisis situation (see Figure 2.1).

Once a crisis has arisen the resulting increase in stress results in a vicious circle with carers and patients' best efforts to cope often compounding the initial disturbance. For this reason almost all crisis intervention strategies are based on stress management. Furthermore, this intervention is most efficient when it is applied at the earliest stage of the crisis. At the earliest warning of a crisis we provide all the resources needed to resolve the crisis, or to prevent escalation to a full-blown episode. This early intervention has been described in Chapter 4. The methods employed are similar and are based upon the principal goal of enhancing the efficiency of the problem-solving efforts of the patient and his or her carers. These strategies will be reviewed briefly, with specific illustrations to show how they are applied during a crisis episode.

Education about the nature of the disorder and clinical management

It will be clear that education is a fundamental aspect of the integrated approach, and is employed at all stages of the person's experience of the disorder. It is essential that adequate information is provided in crisis situations so that the people involved can be clear about the reasons for the behaviour they are experiencing and what is likely to be helpful. Therapists aim to provide the patient and carers with a clear understanding of the nature of the specific mental disorders from which they are suffering. This education focuses on the following issues: diagnosis of the condition through the recognition of characteristic symptom patterns; any immediate changes in stress and vulnerability factors that may be hypothesised as triggering the current crisis (major life events, medication changes, general health and nutritional status); persisting factors that may be sustaining the crisis (unemployment, loss of social supports, noncompliance with medication); analysis of the relative benefits of various specific intervention strategies, including combinations of drug and psychosocial treatments that have specific benefits for key symptom patterns. This discussion attempts to provide realistic expectations of the benefits and costs (both in terms of time and effort as well as unwanted side effects) of the major treatment approaches that the therapy team is advocating.

Education is provided initially in one or more sessions during the first few days of crisis intervention. The precise format of the sessions will be varied according to the capacity of the participants to process information. Usually two or three sessions of 10 to 20 minutes will prove sufficient when accompanied by the use of diagrams, written material and other teaching aids. However, this educational process continues throughout the course of treatment. Wherever possible patient and carers are educated together, so that misunderstanding is minimised. The therapist often finds the patient able to illustrate the nature of the disorder and its treatment much better than any textbook. Furthermore, it is clearly recognised that education is an integrated process, with the therapist gaining understanding whilst facilitating similar understanding among the care group. The integration of the patient and carer into the therapy team is greatly enhanced by this explicit sharing of professional expertise.

Enhancing problem solving efficiency

During the assessment process the therapist clearly acknowledges that the patient and carers have been doing their best to cope with the crisis from their individual perspectives. However, their mutual efforts to cope with a major mental disorder are unlikely to have resulted in all the benefits they would have hoped to have achieved, and at times the coping behaviour of one person may have increased the stress experienced by others. Thus, in order to cope with a crisis in a mental disorder and prevent an escalation of stress in the social environment it is probably necessary to acquire *super-efficient* problem solving skills. Such skills are usually associated with excellent nursing practice, and although many families demonstrate such skills, almost all will benefit from additional coaching and encouragement for their efforts.

When a full-blown crisis has arisen the therapist is expected to become an integral part of the problem-solving unit, and to convene daily problem-solving discussions about everyday stresses, at least until it is clear that the care unit can conduct their own problem solving in a highly efficient manner. Throughout, the therapist encourages the patient and carers to employ their own problem solving. The six-step structured problem-solving method (described in detail in Chapter 7, pp. 212–217) is used at all times, with worksheets completed as records of the discussions. In order to help people to achieve goals in this stressful situation, detailed planning is provided, and therapists provide frequent acknowledgement that seemingly trivial steps become major efforts when a person is acutely disabled with a mental disorder. *Effort* is rewarded rather than *achievement*, and the therapist coaches the patient and carers to carry on their normal roles, rather than supplant their efforts with his or her own coping skills. As the goal is to teach patients and carers skills that they can use throughout the crisis, as well as on future occasions, it is most effective for the therapist to stick with a coaching role as much as po₵ ᵢble. Of course this is not always appropriate, and each plan is negotiated between the therapist and the informal care unit.

The patient's target problems are always addressed, but it is important not to lose sight of the carers' stress problems. Specific issues relating to the carers' needs are given considerable attention. Problem solving is used to develop plans for ensuring that the carers' personal needs for work, recreation, child care, and other interests and commitments are met with minimal disruption or added stress. The carers are trained to monitor their own early warning signs of disorders to which they are prone and are assessed by the therapist on a daily basis.

Monitoring progress

A straightforward method of monitoring progress is devised for each patient and carer. This entails providing a clear chart on which ratings of severity of each targeted problem are recorded on a regular basis by designated raters. These may include the patients, carers or therapists, or a combination of these people. The manner in which the problems are clearly specified facilitates this monitoring process. For example, the number of hours a person sleeps during a 24-hour period can be recorded on a 24-hour sleep chart (Figure 6.6). The quality of each sleep period can be recorded by the patient using a simple coding system. The time a person wakes each morning can be readily seen from the chart. Thus, from one straightforward chart considerably more information can be gleaned than from the question 'How is your sleep?'

Severity of target problems can usually be measured in terms of the frequency or quantity of a specific problem, or in terms of the quality. The quality of a problem may be rated on a simple scale from 0 to 3 (0 = no problem; 1 = mild; 2 = moderate; 3 = severe). Some typical examples of dimensions on which problems may be

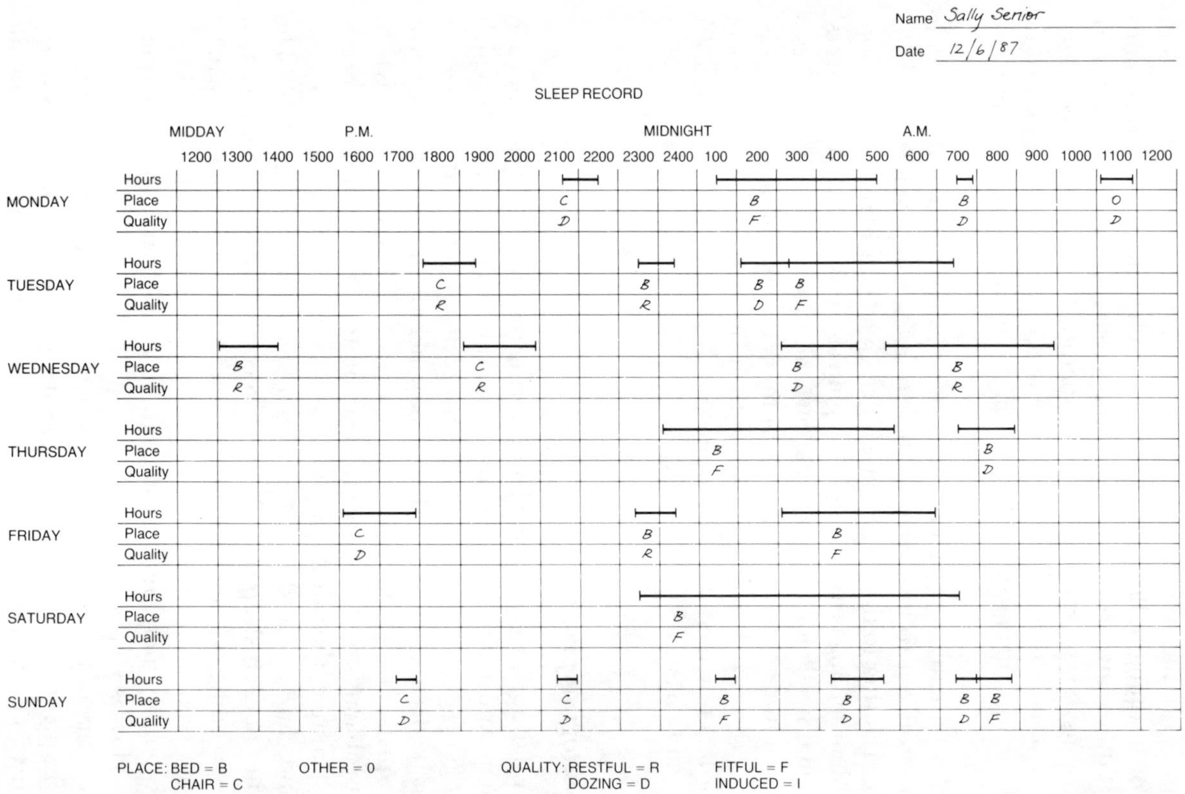

Figure 6.6. A sleep record chart.

Table 6.2. *Dimensions for rating severity of target problems*

Panic attacks	Number per day, severity of each attack
Generalised anxiety	Severity on hourly basis
Depressed mood	Severity on hourly basis
Hallucinations	Frequency, severity of distress associated with each event
Delusions	Severity of preoccupation
Anger	Severity on hourly basis, frequency of aggressive behaviours
Activity levels	Hourly record of specific activities
Agitated behaviours	Hourly record of specified events, severity of subjective feelings
Eating problems	Record of food and drink over 24 hours, record of specific abnormal eating patterns

rated are shown in Table 6.2. In addition to charting changes in the severity of problems, it may be useful to record the manner in which many problems are modified by the context in which they occur. For example, the increase in panic symptoms associated with an attempt to go shopping in a supermarket, would have quite different significance to a similar increase whilst listening to music at home. Similarly, the pattern of disturbance throughout repeated 24-hour observation periods may lead to useful therapeutic insights. For example, we find that sleep charts frequently reveal people with night insomnia actually sleeping their usual 6–8 hours daily, but their pattern of sleep has changed so that they get their most refreshing sleep during the afternoon or early evening, and are frustrated by an inability to sleep during the usual night-time hours. Efforts to increase the total amount of sleep in such cases is usually unrewarding, whereas measures that aim to change the sleep patterns tend to be more successful.

More detailed psychiatric or psychological rating scales are employed to measure changes at a syndrome level on a weekly basis. These are usually interviews accompanied by therapist observations, such as the PSE or Hamilton Scales of Depression or anxiety. These ratings tend to be more global, and are not usually as sensitive measures of change as the specific target ratings of each individual. It is often useful to employ a member of the team other than the key therapist to conduct these ratings in a more objective manner. Additional scales of social functioning and carer burden may be made at this time.

A detailed report on all aspects of progress is provided by the therapist at the weekly meeting of the professional team in the family practice. The entire multidisciplinary team, including the family doctors, meets to review each case, in a manner similar to the hospital ward round. Occasionally patients and carers attend these meetings, but more often the therapist reports progress on their behalf, with the help of their ratings of target problems. However, with severely disturbed people, most members of the team will have contributed to the therapy during the past week and have spent periods in the home. This will include psychiatrists and psychologists, and often the family practitioner as well. Consistent with the overall approach, changes in strategies are made by reviewing specific care plans, redefining problems and goals, and brainstorming alternative solutions using the problem solving approach. Attention is given to the manner in which therapists are coping with the stress of crisis management, and plans derived to support those involved. Above all, praise is given for the *specific efforts* of every team member who has been involved, not merely for outstanding *achievements*.

Training in specific strategies

In addition to the generic stress management approach that we have described above, a variety of strategies are employed to assist with the resolution of specific problems. The efficacy of most of these has been validated in research studies, but a few have been devised from well-established hospital procedures. A selection of those in most common use is summarised here.

Drug strategies

Skilled application of drug strategies is a crucial factor in the effective home-based approach to crisis management of mental disorders. Although it is often concluded that psychoactive drugs have specific therapeutic actions at a syndromal level (e.g. 'antidepressant', 'anxiolytic'), a more discriminating observer may conclude that their action is more specific at a symptom level (i.e. relief of insomnia, reduction of panic, slowing overactive thinking, etc.). Thus, specific drugs are generally targeted to specific symptoms. This approach is one that we have adopted in a more explicit way than is commonly practised. The merits of each drug are considered in terms of the advantages and disadvantages expected in relieving each target problem. For example, the choice of thioridazine to slow the mental and physical overactivity of a person with manic excitement who is reluctant to accept medication may have the advantage of being relatively free of side effects that might lead to non-compliance, but may necessitate taking a large number of tablets, whereas a more potent drug such as haloperidol or fluphenazine may provide the same tranquillising effects with fewer tablets and can also be used in depot preparations, but with the risk of very distressing dystonic reactions. While problem solving of this kind is common in psychiatry, patients themselves and their carers are seldom involved in these discussions, nor indeed are many of the non-medical professional members of the specialist team. In all cases where drugs are considered to have potential value, the choice is a team decision, with the patient making an informed choice, after he or she has been clearly appraised of the expected benefits and risks of particular drugs. The results of treating people in a respectful, collaborative manner tends to reduce the natural tendency to resist that accompanies coercive decision making by professional experts. Such an approach is initially more time consuming, particularly for psychiatrists and family practitioners. However, the long-term benefits of spending up to an hour educating consumers while planning major aspects of their treatment probably outweigh the costs of attempting to deal with the fears of ill-informed people at a later stage.

During an acute exacerbation of symptoms it may be necessary to use more than one drug at a time. However, we attempt to choose one drug only for each target symptom so that polypharmacy is avoided wherever possible. This includes the use of drugs to counter side effects that are dose-related. A simple expedient is to reduce the dose to a level where side effects are less troublesome. Better still, the plasma level of the drug may be assayed, and the drug prescribed within a therapeutic window, such as that necessitated by the high toxicity of lithium salts. Most laboratories can carry out such assays, although the low plasma levels of depot preparations complicate their measurement. The lack of demand for greater scientific precision in the use of psychoactive drugs has led to relatively little understanding of the therapeutic plasma levels of many drugs, despite their extensive morbidity and even mortality. We have found that targeting drugs to specific symptoms and carefully monitoring benefits with specific ratings has contributed to high levels of benefits from many of the most basic and least expensive preparations. Because the integrated management approach does not rely solely on pharmacotherapy, we are able to manage cases with lower doses than those usually recommended for acute disorders. The benefits may develop more slowly, but so do distressing side effects.

Activity schedules

Changes in activity levels are a frequent problem in acute episodes of many mental disorders. Decreased levels of constructive activity are found in depression, anxiety, schizophrenia and mania. However, such changes in constructive activity may be associated with very different overall activity levels. Manic episodes and anxiety may be associated with agitated overactive behaviour and thought patterns, whereas depression and catatonic manifestations of schizophrenia tend to be associated with reduced motor behaviour. In both situations the problem is the reduction in constructive, goal-directed activity. At times disorders may be mixed, with fluctuating activity levels. A simple strategy for managing low levels of constructive activity is *activity scheduling*.

Patients complete a daily record of their main chosen activities on an hour-to-hour basis. They may be requested to make ratings of each activity, such as the pleasure, satisfaction or anxiety they experienced as a result of completing the activity. These records are reviewed with the therapist, who assists the patient and carer to plan and implement a more rewarding pattern of daily activity. People who are frustrated by an inability to perform at their former levels, or to derive similar levels of pleasure from their performance, are helped to break down their efforts into smaller steps they can manage at the present time, and to find ways of maximising their satisfaction and minimising the unpleasant aspects of their daily lives. These efforts to maximise positive feelings and to minimise frustration during crisis periods provide tangible support and serve to reduce the inevitable stress experienced during such episodes.

An example of this was Gary, a 43-year-old businessman, who experienced acute unremitting anxiety. He had waves of panic, could not relax at any time, and was unable to sleep. Any attempt to carry out any activity was interrupted by overwhelming anxiety. He felt desperate and contemplated suicide. His therapist, with the assistance of his wife, recorded his daily activities, and with difficulty he was able to report his level of anxiety while he was engaged in each. It was noticed that he reported less anxiety when engaged, however briefly, in vigorous physical activity, and more anxiety when he attempted sedentary activities, such as watching television or reading. A daily schedule that involved a different physical activity each hour was devised. The activities that Gary chose included walking the dog, chopping firewood, mowing the lawn, hedge cutting, jogging, playing tennis, and taking a walk through the woods with his wife. Problem solving was used to deal with the risk of impulsive self-harm when he was engaged in these activities, and he rehearsed a strategy of stopping the activity immediately, walking away, and carrying out the anxiety management strategies he had been taught. Encouragement for his efforts was provided either by his therapist or his wife, one of whom accompanied him whilst engaged in most of the activities.

After 10 days he found that the time he spent engaged in these activities had increased from 1 hour daily to almost 5 hours. He found that he felt very tired in the evenings and was sleeping several hours (with the added help of a sedative tricyclic drug). He felt moderate satisfaction from his efforts, although remained frustrated that he was missing so much time from his work, and still could not concentrate well enough to engage in even the simplest of business activities. At this stage the therapist suggested that an increase in less physically demanding pleasureable leisure activities might be helpful. These included fishing, visiting a close friend, and playing pool at the local pub.

Anxiety management

Anxiety is a common response to stressful or threatening situations. The combination of intense fear with physiological changes prepares the person to defend themselves or escape from the situation that has triggered the response. In most cases the response far exceeds the real threat from the situation. Harmless insects, animals, social situations, crowds, enclosed spaces and heights may all produce extreme fear. In some cases this may be triggered by thoughts about the future or feelings of inadequacy. In some cases panic may occur in the absence of any clear triggers.

The clinical management of acute episodes of anxiety attempts to help the person identify the precise situations or thoughts that trigger anxiety responses and develop alternative more appropriate responses. This is achieved through a thorough problem analysis followed by the application of those treatments whose effectiveness has been proven (see Chapter 3, pp. 66–71). The integrated approach emphasises education and understanding, and uses a wide range of strategies including: reduction in intake of stimulants such as tea, coffee and stimulant prescription and non-prescription drugs; desensitisation to feared situations or thoughts; relaxation exercises; respiratory control; behaviour rehearsal; and distraction. At times of crisis, people may have difficulty recalling strategies which they had previously employed successfully. Attention is therefore often focussed on helping the person to recall and utilise these skills. Demonstration by the therapist (modelling) accompanied by the patient's rehearsal of the strategy facilitates the application of many strategies.

Persistent negative thinking

Unpleasant thoughts tend to predominate in almost all florid episodes of mental disorders, with the exception of manic states. In recent years considerable advances have been made in the development of cognitive strategies that aim to modify such thought processes and to direct them into more constructive patterns. The best known of these approaches have been those pioneered by Beck and his colleagues (Beck et al, 1979). The reader is referred to this work for further details.

Among the strategies that prove most useful in florid episodes are those that help the individual pinpoint the realistic problem issues associated with their persistent negative thoughts and to use the problem-solving method to devise alternative plans to tackle these issues. For example, a man who felt profound remorse for having 'stolen' a family relic at the time his family estate was being dispersed after the death of his mother, was able to devise and then carry out a plan that involved confessing his misdemeanour to his elder sister, who immediately forgave him. He stopped worrying about this issue, and experienced some relief from his guilt-ridden thinking.

Effective reassurance

Training carers (and professionals) to provide effective reassurance is of major importance in the management of many anxiety and depressive states. The tendency to tell people that they will be alright, or the situation is not as bad as they think, seldom provides sufferers with the support they seek. A more effective method is to take the time to discuss their key concerns in a problem-solving framework that addresses the issues fully, with the opportunity for clear action plans, that when implemented, may be expected to provide tangible benefits for the patient. Regularly scheduled problem-solving sessions of this kind enable carers and professionals to respond to persistent requests for reassurance with the firm commitment that this concern will be discussed in full at the next problem-solving session.

Sleep management

Disturbed sleep is probably the most frequent target symptom in acute crises. It may take various forms – difficulty getting off to sleep, difficulty staying asleep, waking too early, not getting enough sleep, sleeping too much, nightmares and restless sleep. One additional problem for home-based management is that disturbed sleep of one person tends to affect the entire household, particularly those sharing the same bedroom. The lack of sleep of carers is one of the commonest complaints that contributes to their burnout. Furthermore, a refreshing night's sleep is one of the most potent therapeutic factors for all mental health problems. Thus, it is crucial that sleep patterns are restored at an early stage in the crisis.

In addition to problem solving with the care unit, the following strategies are useful in assisting with specific issues:

completing a sleep chart (see Figure 6.6)
review of caffeine and other stimulant intake and reduce to minimal levels
review of sedative intake, including alcohol, antihistamines and other non-prescription sedatives
review of all prescription drugs for sedative/stimulant, suppression of REM sleep patterns, etc
review of physical complaints, especially pain, cramps, etc.
education of patient and carers about sleep – dispel the eight hours per night myth; restrict sleeping to a comfortable bed; consider temporary separate beds/rooms for partners (although sexual activity may benefit sleep); planning constructive activities to carry on without disturbing others
self-hypnosis through deep muscle relaxation and cognitive strategies

prescription of sedative drugs targeted to the specific type of disturbance

As well as the sleep chart, specific handouts are used for education about sleep and relaxation training. At times audiotaped instructions may help with self hypnosis, but the patient must acquire a recorder that switches itself off when the play back has finished.

Managing disorders of eating

The problem-solving method that we employ necessitates a clearly specified formulation of the specific problem behaviours, with their associated cognitions and emotional states. Although certain patterns of eating have been considered deviant and have been labelled anorexia nervosa or bulimia, problems with appropriate nutrition are frequent in most mental disorders. The most common problem presenting as a crisis is low caloric intake associated with appetite reduction and excessive weight loss. Such a problem is found in depression, generalised anxiety, obsessive compulsive disorders as well as the specific eating disorders. People suffering from persecutory ideas may refuse food if they believe it has been poisoned. Overeating less often presents as a crisis, although excessive fluid intake may prove fatal as a result of water intoxication, excessive caffeine intake may contribute to insomnia, and of course the problems of excessive alcohol are well known, and are commonly associated with inadequate nutrition.

Comprehensive assessment includes monitoring with daily intake charts, that describe the psychosocial context as well as the actual food consumed, questionnaires about attitudes associated with eating, such as the Eating Attitudes Test (Garner & Garfinkel, 1979), patient and carers' problem-solving efforts, and a weekly weight chart. The frequent association between physical illness and appetite and weight loss should never be overlooked and the family practitioner should once again ensure that underlying physical disorders are assessed and treated.

A baseline assessment is conducted, preferably over a period of at least one week, before any specific strategies are applied. Once again the clinical management plan is based upon the specific contingencies that surround each particular case. The therapist attempts to construct a plan that builds on the existing efforts of patient and carers to overcome the problem. The goal of therapy will be the establishment of a healthy eating pattern that maintains adequate nutrition. A number of specific strategies that may be employed to this end are summarised:

education about nutrition, including accepted weight ranges for each person

contracted agreement on schedules for food intake that involve patient, carers and therapists

self-monitoring; handing responsibility back to the patient wherever feasible, with choice of foods, etc.

specific rewards for adherence to agreed eating behaviours, these are agreed as part of the contract between patient, carers and therapists

attempts to stimulate appetite through choice and preparation of foods the patient still enjoys

use of caloric supplements, particularly if preferred by the patient

enhancing the aspects of meals that patient specifically enjoys

providing longer time periods for persons with retardation to complete their meals, and assisting carers to spend time relaxing with them during these prolonged meal times

avoiding coercive strategies and threats; as ever, *provide encouragement for effort not achievement;* shape appropriate behaviour in small steps

anxiety management, where food ingestion is accompanied by high levels of anxiety, or obsessional behaviours

cognitive-behavioural strategies to deal with irrational beliefs and assumptions that are not ameliorated by education

pharmacotherapy – to date no drugs have demonstrated consistent appetite stimulating effects, although sedative tricyclic drugs such as amitriptyline and chlomipramine appear to facilitate weight gain in people with anorexia associated with other depressive symptoms

The manner in which several strategies are integrated into a treatment plan is illustrated by the following case example:

Mary was a 56-year-old woman, who co-managed a farm with her husband. She suffered recurrent depressive episodes that were characterised by marked anorexia and sleep disturbance with depressed mood and guilt feelings.

A problem analysis of her eating behaviour revealed that she lacked appetite for starchy foods and most meats, but retained a small appetite for fruit juices and light salads and lightly cooked vegetables. She drank 2–3 mugs of tea per day. She felt full after two or three mouthfuls, but would continue to eat slowly if not pressured. Any coercion triggered feelings of guilt about people starving in the developing countries and further reduced her minimal desire to eat. Left to her own devices she would not eat at all. Her husband, Frank, encouraged her to eat regular meals, but without Mary's usual enthusiasm for food and excellent cooking, he too tended to skip meals and merely prepare tinned and frozen foods, sitting down to eat in front of television with a tray, rather than at the kitchen table as usual. Mary had lost eight pounds in the past six weeks and continued to lose about two pounds a week. She remained moderately overweight.

Problem solving with the couple developed the following initial plan:

1 Frank to assist Mary to plan a menu for each day the evening before and to write it down on a chart
2 Frank to assist Mary with food preparation. Focus on salads with fruits, nuts, cheese and diced meats or canned tuna or salmon.
3 Therapist to take Mary to purchase a cookery book on interesting salads.
4 Eat at the table at lunch and dinner. Both cleanly dressed. And talk about everyday events.
5 Therapist to be present at lunch each day to coach Frank and Mary, especially how to support Mary's eating behaviour and demonstrate how to distract Mary from her guilt feelings.
6 Therapist to stay until Mary has completed her meal so that Frank can get back to work within an hour.
7 Mary to complete simple chart of what she ate and drank.

The review at the end of the first week of implementation showed that the plan was partially successful. Some progress had been made with all steps, although Mary had eaten only half the food she had aimed to, and had lost a further two pounds. She had, however, been less distressed by guilt feelings at mealtimes and was clearly trying to eat as much as she felt able. Her fluid intake was adequate and she sipped orange juice regularly to counter the dry mouth she experienced as a result of the tricyclic drug she was taking for her sleep disturbance. The therapist coached Frank to change the subject to an every day discussion about the farm whenever Mary made guilt-ridden or otherwise negative comments that could not be problem solved. He conducted two 20-minute sessions with Frank on his own to rehearse this strategy. At first Frank found this difficult, until he realised that his attempts to empathise with Mary merely contributed to her becoming increasingly distressed, rather than reassured. The therapist highlighted the small, but specific steps that had been achieved by both partners and praised them warmly for their efforts.

During the following three weeks Mary's appetite gradually returned and meals became more pleasant and relaxed events, with the therapist spending less time with them at lunchtimes. It was important for the therapist to maintain a therapeutic coaching role rather than a social role in this situation.

Traditional barriers are often eroded as the family becomes part of the therapeutic team. In many instances therapists will eat meals with families. However, just as with meetings in the workplace, distinctions are made between social lunch hours and working lunch meetings. The same sort of distinctions serve to clarify functions when working with people at home. Handling issues, such as how family members respond to unexpected visitors arriving during therapeutic sessions, or how to introduce the therapists to friends they meet when out shopping, need to be problem solved with the family so that embarrassment is minimised. On the whole we have found that the greater exposure of mental health professionals in this humanistic way has led to improved community awareness and reduction of stigma for patients and their carers. Further discussion about these issues is provided in Chapter 10.

Managing delusions, paranoid ideas and hallucinations

Neuroleptic drugs have made a major impact on the control of psychotic phenomena. This has enabled many people to reside in unrestricted settings, and acute episodes to be treated at home. However, 25% of people who experience these symptoms do not respond to drug therapy and continue to experience severe disturbance. A number of strategies have been developed that supplement the benefits achieved by drugs. Few of these methods have been validated by replicated controlled trials. Thus, their application must always be regarded as experimental and this should be made clear to patients and carers. However, they are usually eager to try a new idea when their own efforts to cope effectively with the disturbance have failed. Some of the strategies that have been described as effective in case studies include:

Problem solving: Rather than confront the irrational beliefs directly, carers invite the patient to discuss the idea within a problem solving framework. This facilitates discussion of alternative explanations for the belief in a non-judgmental atmosphere, as well as developing consistent responses to expressions of the belief. Carers learn the futility of arguing with a person's belief system, and that alternatives such as simply stating their views in a non-emotive fashion, tend to work better than taking a forceful advocacy position.

Defining the contingencies that trigger delusions and hallucinations: A careful problem analysis may uncover the specific biobehavioural setting in which these psychotic experiences may be most likely to occur for each individual. A wide range of circumstances may be found. One person may feel persecuted when in crowded places, another when he is alone and feels abandoned. One person may hear voices when relaxing, another when highly excited, and so on. It may help to have a cooperative person keep a continuous record of the settings in which their targeted symptoms occur. This may include the place, activity, thoughts and feelings. The sophistication of this self-monitoring will depend on the person's cognitive capacity at the time, but it is often surprising how well many severely disabled people can carry out this task. Where the contingencies that trigger or maintain a symptom can be pinpointed, it is possible for the person to modify the specific elements that appear to contribute. One person found he became very tense and held his breath just before he heard a voice. He learned to relax himself at this time and to take several slow deep breaths, and found that he had fewer unpleasant hallucinations. Another person with persecutory ideas tried to avoid any eye contact with people by staring at the ground when he walked in the street, but then felt convinced that everybody was looking at him and whispering derogatory comments (some indeed were, according to his wife). He agreed to try the opposite and to look at every passer by. This eased the tension considerably, although he still believed that a group of people were conspiring to kill him, particularly those who looked back and smiled at him.

Thought stopping: This technique has been applied with success in a few cases of people with delusions and hallucinations. The person learns to shout stop under his or her breath when preoccupied by a delusion or hallucination. They then attempt to change the theme of their thoughts to a specific pleasant subject. The addition of a self-administered mild aversive stimulus, such as flicking a rubber band against one's wrist may assist this strategy.

We have used these various strategies and have found that people obtain considerable relief once they manage to achieve at least partial control of these distressing experiences.

Anger control

The threat of violence is one of the major public concerns many people express about caring for people experiencing acute episodes of mental disorders at home. Despite reassurance that surveys indicate that people suffering from mental disorders are no more violent than any other members of the community, the excessive media attention generated by the occasional violent mentally disordered offender, has created a major stigma that is difficult to overcome. Carers are understandably concerned that a person who has irrational thoughts may unexpectedly carry out unprovoked acts of aggression against them. When a person is acutely disordered the risk of aggression is indeed increased. However, such behaviour is seldom unprovoked, rather, the provocation at these times may be much less than at other times when the person's mental state is more stable. Thus, the management of anger differs little with mental disorders than in other situations.

As with all targeted problems, the first approach is to conduct a thorough problem analysis. This helps establish the most likely situations where aggressive actions may occur, and also highlights the ways in which a person and social environment is controlling angry impulses already. As with most problems the solutions are often already being applied and the therapist merely facilitates their more efficient application by structuring these informal efforts in to a well-planned program. It is important to look at those occasions where angry impulses are controlled and to contrast them with occasions where aggression has resulted.

The principles of anger control that we have employed include the following:

Education that anger is a natural emotion that cannot be avoided or effectively suppressed.

The appropriate expression of anger often assists in resolving problems and achieving goals.

Each person must take full responsibility for the origins of their own feelings and not blame other people's actions for *causing* their unpleasant emotional states.

Aggressive acts can never be excused, even when the person acts under extreme provocation – there is always an alternative to violence.

Assaults on persons or property are illegal. They should always be reported to the police, who should take responsibility for ensuring that legal procedures are adhered to according to the laws agreed by the community in which the offender resides. A mental disorder does not exonerate any citizen from any law or the appropriate legal processes. It may affect the type of sentence given to an offender at the completion of a trial. Mental health professionals should only advocate 'treatments' that have been validated as effective in preventing recidivism associated with a specific misdemeanour.

Carers are also likely to experience angry feelings towards the mentally disordered person. Efforts to ensure that they too express their anger appropriately may prove crucial. Some stress reduction measures appear to advocate suppression of all expression of negative feelings towards the index patient. While this may be of limited value at the time of florid episodes in some cases, it has potential hazards for the carers if continued.

The clear aim of anger control is the *appropriate expression* of strong angry feelings within a problem-solving framework. This involves the following skills:

Pinpointing exactly what has triggered the angry feeling. This is often some aspect of a person's behaviour or a specific context, e.g. a threatening gesture; a remark or action perceived as rejecting or belittling; a crowded place; feeling cornered, etc. Of course such cues may be amplified by negative thought patterns, persecutory ideas or hallucinations.

Deciding whether immediate expression of the angry feeling will lead to efficient resolution, and reduce the likelihood of its recurrence, or will it probably escalate tension.

Tell the person who is the target of your expression exactly what they have done that has triggered off your anger. If this is their own behaviour stick to that one specific behaviour and avoid broadening the discussion to other less relevant behaviour or issues. In other words, *target the problem, not the person!*

Tell them exactly how you feel in that situation, using appropriate non-verbal expression; e.g. eye contact, firm tone of voice. Avoid aggressive postures such as standing over a person and crowding them, or threatening gestures, raised voice, or sarcasm.

Try to suggest some ways that the person could modify their behaviour in future that would prevent your angry response. If necessary, be prepared to carry out a longer problem-solving discussion using the six-step method (see pp. 212–215).

This method of expressing negative feelings is identical to that employed in the communication skills training that is a major component of the approach that we employ to assist patients and their carers to manage stress (see pp. 211–212). It can be employed to express any feeling in a clear, direct manner.

It is clear that learning to communicate anger in a non-aggressive way may take some time, and that with the extreme provocation that many mental disorders engender, added strategies may be needed as interim contingencies. Two useful strategies are limit setting and time out.

Limit setting   This strategy involves negotiating with the potentially aggressive person the precise behaviours that will be tolerated by household members, and the precise behaviours that will not. This definition of limits forms part of the contract for community-based treatment (see p. 164). The immediate response to an unacceptable aggressive action is also agreed between the parties. This usually involves removing the offender immediately from the household circle, but in keeping with our overall approach, the precise plan is left to the discretion of the patient and carers. However, we advocate taking a very strong line on any form of violence or emotional abuse, and urge people to do likewise, if necessary assisting them to call in police or other social agencies at an early stage. Good rapport with the local police may facilitate visits from a police officer to clarify the legal consequences of such acts to a potential offender in a firm yet understanding manner. The police may need to rehearse this performance to ensure they convey the message in the appropriate manner. However, it is our experience that police officers have excellent skills in expression of limit setting. This clear support assists carers who may hesitate to call the police in an emergency situation. It is crucial that any specified example of inappropriate behaviour is managed according to the contract. Many people tend to dismiss minor offences, thereby reinforcing them and increasing the likelihood that they will escalate to major offences. A consistent approach to setting limits is a very valuable strategy in the prevention of violence.

Time out   Many people will be familiar with the use of time out in parenting. However, when the offender is an adult it is not a simple task to frog-march them to the bathroom and have them remain there for a specified time. A variant that has proved useful with adults involves the same principle of removing the person from the provoking situation and withdrawing positive reinforcement for inappropriate behaviour. A contract is agreed that when clear warning signs appear that are prodromes of an aggressive act the person is prompted to leave the situation immediately and carry out some behaviour that is likely to reduce the risk of aggression. Commonly this involves prompting the person to take a walk or engage in some physical activity that helps them unwind. Patients are encouraged to recognise the warning signs themselves and to initiate this behaviour themselves to assist their self-control. Once again in order to prove effective this approach must be clearly specified and applied in a highly consistent manner. Therapists may rehearse the situation several times with patient and carers. In addition, it is useful to rehearse likely snags in its application, and problem solve how they may be handled.

A final cautionary note involves the use of drugs to promote anger control. To date there have been no drugs developed that show a consistent anti-aggressive effect. However, it is common for doctors to consider that this is one benefit associated with tranquillising drugs. It is not our policy to use any drug as a means of behaviour control. Rather we are eager to ensure that drug and psychological strategies are employed only in the clinical management of those specific impairments for which there is adequate scientific evidence for their specific efficacy. Thus, we would use a tranquillising drug to reduce the perceptual disturbance that results in hallucinations and delusions or to slow manic thought processes, all of which may predispose a person to aggressive acts. Overenthusiastic prescribing of high doses of drugs may have the paradoxical effect of reducing self-control over violent impulses or of producing toxic confusional states where the risk of violence is heightened (Curry et al, 1970).

Managing suicide risk

Suicide is another form of behaviour that has a very low frequency of occurrence, yet is a major concern for mental health professionals. The ability to forestall suicide attempts and their resulting fatalities has been considered a key measure of the success of a community-based mental health service.

A person suffering from a major mental disorder, particularly depressive episodes, schizophrenia or severe persistent anxiety states has a higher risk of suicide than a mentally healthy member of the community. In addition, alcoholism and major stress, especially bereavement, work failure and marital breakdown where loss is profound, carry a similarly increased risk. Reliable methods of determining this risk have yet to be formulated, and current studies have shown how difficult it is to predict the specific individuals who will commit suicide. Nevertheless a review of the literature enabled us to devise a checklist of risk factors (see Table 4.2). Whenever a person is suspected of having thoughts of suicide or self-destruction therapists conduct a tactful and comprehensive screening that aims to develop rapport and trust, while displaying concern about current life problems. The assessment enabled the checklist to be completed. If six or more items are checked as present the suicide risk is considered 'high' regardless of expressed threats or other evidence of self-destructive intentions. The following procedures are applied without delay:

1. Therapist consults with a psychiatrist.
2. Ensure that the high risk person is appropriately supervised at all times of the day and night by a carer who fully comprehends the danger and is willing to take responsibility for monitoring the person's behaviour.
3. In the absence of people both capable *and willing* to undertake this monitoring responsibility, a mental health professional(s) must be assigned to carry out this task. This may necessitate admission to a hospital unit.
4. Access to potential suicide weapons is reduced in a firm, yet diplomatic way. This includes removal of all sharp knives, razors and guns, all unused drugs, alcohol supplies, and dangerous chemicals.
5. Drugs are prescribed in small doses by the family practitioner, and a clear note is made on the front of the chart to alert other doctors to current concerns. At times all doctors covering the practice need to be informed of these concerns.
6. A written contract was drawn up in close collaboration with the high-risk person and carers, stating that he or she will agree to contact a specific person or agency before performing any self-destructive actions. This states clearly the services that will be provided to assist the person through the current crisis. The person at risk is requested to sign this statement, which is then

countersigned by the key therapist. This contract is left with the
person, a copy is made for his carer, a copy for his family
practitioner, and a copy for the mental health service.

7. Suicidal intention is reassessed using the hopelessness scale of
   the Hamilton Rating Scale for Depression and standardised
   questions from the PSE on a daily basis until risk becomes
   minimal.

8. Clinical management of underlying disorder or dysfunction
   begins without delay.

9. The Checklist is used only a rough guide of suicide risk factors.
   Every case is treated on its merits, and distressed persons are
   encouraged to seek help from the mental health team or other
   professionals on a 24-hour basis.

10. All threats of self-destructive actions are treated as potential
    antecedents of such actions, regardless of the manner in which
    they are communicated.

In summary, the key elements of suicide prevention we employ are
comprehensive assessment, effective monitoring of risk factors, and
application of effective treatment of the underlying problems, both
psychosocial and biological. Consistent with our approach patients
and their carers are considered at the centre of all clinical management and their efforts to cope with the crisis were always integrated
with those of the professional services.

References

Beck A.T., Rush A.J., Shaw B.F. & Emery G. (1979) *Cognitive therapy of
   depression.* Guilford Press, New York.
Clare, A. (1976) *Psychiatry in dissent.* Tavistock, London.
Curry S.H., Marshall J.H.L., Davis J.S. & Janowsky D.J. (1970)
   Chlorpromazine plasma levels and effects. *Archives of General
   Psychiatry,* **22**, 289–296.
Falloon I.R.H., Mueser K., Gingerich S., Rappaport S., McGill C. &
   Hole V. (1988) *Behavioural family therapy: a workbook.* Buckingham
   Mental Health Service, Buckingham, UK.
Falloon I.R.H. & Talbot R.E. (1981) Persistent auditory hallucinations.
   Coping mechanisms and implications for management. *Psychological
   Medicine,* **11**, 329–339.
Fenton F.R., Tessier L., Struening E.L., Smith F.A. & Benoit C. (1981)
   Home and hospital psychiatric treatment. Croom Helm, London.

Garner D.M. & Garfinkel P.E. (1979) The Eating Attitude Test: an index of the symptoms of anorexia nervosa. *Psychological Medicine*, **9**, 273–279.

Goffman E. (1961) *Asylums*. Anchor Books, New York.

Hoult J. (1986) Community care for the acutely mentally ill. *British Journal of Psychiatry*, **149**, 137–144.

Langsley D. G., Flomenhaft K. & Matchotka P. (1971) Avoiding mental hospital admission: a follow-up study. *American Journal of Psychiatry*, **127**, 1391–1394.

Mosher L.R. & Burti L. (1989) *Community mental health practice*. Norton, New York.

Muijen M., Marks I.M., Connolly J., Audini B. & McNamee G. (1992) The Daily Living Program. Preliminary comparison of community versus hospital-based treatment the severely mentally ill facing emergency admission. *British Journal of Psychiatry*, **160**, 379–384.

Scott R.D. (1974) Cultural frontiers in the mental health service. *Schizophrenia Bulletin*, **10**, 58–73.

Stein L.I. & Test M.A. (1976) Retraining hospital staff to work in a community program in Wisconsin. *Hospital and Community Psychiatry*, **27**, 266–268.

Stein L.I. & Test M.A. (1980) Alternative to the mental hospital. I. Conceptual model, treatment program and clinical evaluation. *Archives of General Psychiatry*, **37**, 392–397.

Test M.A., Knoedler W. & Allness D. (1985) The long-term treatment of young schizophrenics in a community support program. In L.I. Stein & M.A. Test (Eds.) *The training in community living model: a decade of experience*. New directions in mental health services, No. 26. Jossey-Bass, San Francisco.

Test M A. & Stein L.I. (1980) Alternative to the mental hospital treatment. III. Social cost. *Archives of General Psychiatry*, **37**, 409–412.

Vaughn C.E. & Leff J.P. (1976) The measurement of expressed emotion in families of psychiatric patients. *British Journal of Social and Clinical Psychology*, **15**, 157–165

Weisbrod B.A., Test M.A. & Stein L.I. (1980) Alternative to the mental hospital. II. Economic cost-benefit analysis. *Archives of General Psychiatry*, **37**, 400–405.

Wing J.K., Cooper J.E. & Sartorius N. (1974) *The measurement and classification of psychiatric symptoms*. Cambridge University Press, Cambridge.

7

Prevention of recurrent disorders

An effective service aims not merely to facilitate recovery from florid episodes of mental disorders, but also to ensure that the risk of future recurrent episodes is minimised. As with other aspects of integrated care the vulnerability–stress model of mental disorders underpins the approach to prevention of recurrence of mental disorders (see Figure 2.1, p. 29). It is assumed that recurrent episodes are most likely when either a person's biological vulnerability increases, and/or environmental stress overwhelms his or her current coping capacity. Relatively little is known about the fluctuations in biological vulnerability, apart from the diurnal variations in adrenal hormones and the female menstrual cycle. The latter appears to be frequently associated with re-emergence of symptoms of mental disorders. Other biological influences, such as nutritional variables, the effects of concurrent physical disorders, brain damage, and the toxic effects of various prescription and illicit drugs have been implicated in recurrence of florid episodes of many mental disorders. However, it seems reasonable to assume that fluctuations in biological vulnerability occur and that these factors are not constant.

The role of stress factors in triggering episodes of disorders is at a similarly primitive state of understanding. A series of studies on household stress has suggested that the risk of recurrence is most likely where a person spends a substantial amount of time in contact with persons who provoke interpersonal stress (Falloon,, 1988), and that risk is lowered when vulnerable persons spend a greater proportion of their time associating with more supportive individuals. Very little is understood about stress at work or leisure. However, again it seems likely that coercive relationships tend to provoke recurrent episodes, whereas interpersonal support reduces this risk (Wing et al, 1964). Psychological factors such as persistent negative thinking and low self-esteem have been considered to increase the vulnerability to recurrent episodes of depressive disorders (Beck et al, 1978).

The occurrence of life events that provoke major stress appears to precede recurrent episodes of schizophrenic, anxiety and manic disorders more frequently than one would expect if this was a chance association (Paykel, 1978). One study has suggested that recurrent episodes of schizophrenia may be provoked either by high levels of ambient stress or the occurrence of a major life event (Leff and Vaughn,, 1981). A major life event is one that causes ongoing moderate or severe stress. Events such as a death of a close associate, break up of an important relationship, loss of a job or moving house are usually considered major events. However, each person perceives stress idiosyncratically, and what is stressful to one person may not be percieved as such by another. It is therefore important to define the stressor in terms of how much stress it causes each individual (Brown & Harris, 1978). For this reason assessment of stress is a complex task and standardised measures are cumbersome and beyond the resources of most clinical services. Simpler versions such as the Vulnerability–Stress Checklist (see p. 300) that we have employed have no scientific validation, but may help to alert therapists of the need to review a wide range of factors in their ongoing assessments of people's needs.

Research studies suggest that stress does not have a direct effect on a disorder, rather environmental stress induces physiological changes that add to existing biological vulnerability to a disorder. This is a non-specific change that differs widely among individuals. Whereas one person may experience raised blood pressure, another may experience an increase in muscle tension, and still another an increase in gastric acid production.

Physiological changes may or may not parallel psychological awareness of stress and consequent coping responses. A person who recognises that he or she is experiencing excess stress may be able to initiate action to cope effectively with the stress-provoking situation. Lack of awareness of the effects of stress may prevent early response. However, with most disorders there is a further intermediate step before a recurrence of their disorder eventuates. The physiological responses are associated with symptoms such as headaches, appetite loss, sleep disturbance and feelings of apprehension. Such symptoms are non-specific, but are highly consistent for each individual over time, so that they can be readily recognised by the sufferer and serve as warning signs of excess stress and the need for immediate steps to cope with the underlying stress that has provoked them. With some disorders the time between the onset of stress and the onset of a florid episode is relatively long; in the case of depressive disorders this period may be several months; in others, such as mania, the delay may be no more than 24 hours. This poses a problem for devising strategies to assist the person in countering the effects of stress. In some cases it is critical to ensure that stress is resolved with minimal delay, in others such urgent attention may be somewhat less important. Of course when people have experienced previous episodes of a disorder, these time factors are usually consistent and the response can be tailored to each person's different needs.

In summary, we have assumed that biological and environmental factors interact continually and that recurrences of mental disorders can often be predicted when patterns of both forms of stressor can be defined for individuals. When a threshold is exceeded the vulnerable person is placed at a higher risk of having a florid episode. The longer this threshold is exceeded, the greater the likelihood of an episode. Our approach entails devising strategies that enable persons to counter the effects of stress of all kinds and to minimise the time period over which their stress threshold is exceeded, thereby protecting themselves from significant exacerbations of their conditions. This prophylaxis is provided by integrating five main interventions:

1 Targeted prophylactic drug therapy.
2 Education about mental disorders.
3 Detecting early warning signs.
4 Training in efficient stress management.
5 Social case work.

Targeted prophylactic drug therapy

The benefits of continuing to take drugs after a florid episode has passed has proved effective for schizophrenic, depressive and manic disorders (Davis et al, 1980; Prien et al, 1984; Schou, 1989). The benefits in reduction of the risk of recurrence are greatest for schizophrenia, with less dramatic, but nonetheless clinically

Table 7.1. *Compliance management*

EXPECT poor adherence
Involve carers throughout
Educate about benefits and costs
Self-monitor benefits and costs
Collaborate on targeting optimal doses throughout
Plan strategies to cope with unwanted effects
Train drug-taking habits
Specific rewards for adherence
Early detection of cognitive dysfunction/recurrence
Problem solving for reduced adherence

significant evidence to support their continuation in the major affective disorders. Two major problems limit the benefits of long-term drug prophylaxis. These are, inadequate adherence to the recommended dose regimens, and the development of unpleasant side effects. Several strategies have been devised that aim to counter these drawbacks.

Establishing and maintaining adherence to long-term drug regimens

Very few people welcome the prospect of taking drugs on a continuing basis after the florid manifestations of their disorders have abated. Thus it is not surprising that the majority of drugs recommended for ingestion by psychiatric outpatients are not taken (Soskis, 1978). The success of drug therapy in the community will be determined largely by the levels of compliance achieved. Considerable effort therefore is directed towards achieving adherence to drug regimens (Table 7.1). It is crucial to realise that taking medication is a complex cognitive-behavioural response that must be learned by the patient and his or her carers. The process by which a person learns habitual drug taking may be interfered with by a large number of environmental contingencies. On the other hand the prescribing physician may facilitate this learning process by employing a number of relatively straightforward strategies. The following steps described below are considered for every case.

A problem analysis of drug taking

In order to achieve adequate compliance a careful review of the current drug-taking patterns of each person is an important first step. It must be assumed that everyone will comply poorly at times. The therapist helps the patient define the contingencies that surround both good and poor compliance. Although the drug-taking patterns of individuals will differ greatly, a number of issues frequently lead to poor compliance. These problems are discussed below along with several strategies that may help to resolve them.

Attendance for clinic appointments   When drugs are provided at outpatient clinics there may be a high rate of non-attendance. Parkes and co-workers (1962) noted that non-attendance for initial outpatient appointments after recovery from a florid episode was the most common reason for failure to establish regular drug taking. There are many reasons for this, from obvious practical matters, such as lack of instructions on how to get to the clinic, loss of appointment cards, concern about taking time off work, to more complex issues, such as a lack of understanding of the rationale for continuation of therapy, or anxiety about attending a psychiatric clinic and spending long periods waiting in crowded rooms. The need to improve administrative procedures, to provide a clear rationale for therapy, to minimise waiting, and to make clinics more welcoming may reduce the practical problems. But some people will need anxiety management to overcome the fear of sitting in a waiting room, and everyone seems to benefit from education about the benefits of continuing drug therapy and the risks of not doing so.

The provision of drugs by the person's family practitioner at the family practice clinic is helpful, particularly when appointments are available outside working hours. The addition of an outreach service to provide drugs for patients at their homes may assist those who remain too disorganised to attend clinics. However, this arrangement is unlikely to improve the compliance of patients who refuse to accept the value of drugs and elect to remain drug free.

Forgetfulness   Perhaps the most common cause of poor compliance is forgetfulness. This problem is amplified by the presence of cognitive disorganisation found in florid phases of most mental disorders. This problem is further compounded by the unwillingness of most hospitals to train patients to take tablets when they are inpatients. Training in self-administration, or the training of carers to administer tablets to persistently disorganised people, is essential to ensure maintenance of adequate compliance.

Other strategies that may help include simplification of the tablet-taking regimen to a once-daily dose, or linking tablet taking to a well-established habit, such as mealtimes, bathing or brushing teeth. Training those who regularly brush their teeth before retiring to bed to place their daily dose of tablets next to their toothpaste has assisted many to establish regular ingestion. This also provides carers with an unobtrusive way of checking that the tablets have been taken.

Some people find that keeping a week's supply of tablets in a plastic container divided into subsections for each day helps them remember which tablets are to be taken and at what times. This is particularly helpful for the person who moves about and has to take tablets when away from home. Some drug companies have developed standard packaging along these lines. Unfortunately dose variation makes this somewhat impractical.

Consistent with our model of minimally sufficient response to problems, we suggest that it is preferable for people to take responsibility for their own tablet taking. Nagging by concerned carers is usually counterproductive. However, training carers in effective prompting and rewarding of adherence to drug taking may be highly beneficial.

Unpleasant side effects   The high prevalence of unpleasant side effects associated with most psychoactive drugs is considered a major factor in reduced compliance. The psychomotor effects of akathisia and akinesia have been most clearly linked to poor compliance of neuroleptics, and the anticholinergic effects of dry mouth and drowsiness have been implicated in reduced adherence to antidepressant drugs. While a person may feel inclined to persevere despite these unpleasant effects when they are experiencing distressing symptoms, the benefits become comparatively less as the florid symptoms remit, and consequently motivation to continue is reduced. A self-administered trial of the drugs is likely to relieve the unpleasant effects and provide further support for discontinuing the drug. Thus, it is crucial to anticipate such events and to ensure that all reported side effects are minimised at all times, and that patients and their carers are clearly educated about the benefits and risks of the drugs they are being asked to take. It is also essential for the therapist to encourage patients and carers to be open about whether or not the patient is continuing to take medication regularly and to discuss any difficulties. Any problems are addressed in a problem-solving manner with further education frequently being provided. By dealing with difficulties in this way we seemed to avoid the situation where people are afraid to disclose their non-compliance to their therapist. In addition, several strategies have been shown to help people to cope with common side effects:

Do nothing: because side effects are usually maximal soon after starting a drug and tend to diminish with time, patients are encouraged to continue to take medication regularly until the unpleasant effects subside.

Dose reduction: most side effects are related directly to the dose of the drug. Reduction in the dose will usually result in a reduction of side effects. Almost all drugs have a prophylactic effect at lower doses than those used to control florid symptoms. Thus, physicians are encouraged to collaborate with patients to find the minimum effective dose.

Self-regulation: patients are discouraged from self-regulation, unless this is part of a plan worked out with their doctors. Many side effects are made worse by variations in daily dose. However, some patients are able to learn to adjust their doses to provide optimal efficacy on a day-by-day basis. Careful monitoring of the stress levels and the detection of prodromal phases of florid episodes has enabled many patients who have experienced schizophrenic episodes to target their drug prophylaxis specifically to those periods of high stress or impending recurrence and to remain free of the burdens of continual drug-taking at other times. A variation of this targeted approach involves taking very low doses continually and increasing the dose when an episode threatens. Both these approaches tend to produce more frequent minor episodes, but with benefits associated with fewer side effects.

Change drug: there is a wide range of drugs with proven efficacy for prevention of any disorder. Despite similar benefits, their side effects profiles tend to differ. The physician is usually able to select a drug that has a side effect profile that proves least distressing for each individual.

Drugs to counter side effects: a variety of drugs have been used to counter the unpleasant effects of neuroleptic drugs. Of course these drugs have their own range of side effects, and have been shown to have maximal benefits during the first few weeks they are taken.

Non-drug strategies: the problems associated with side effects can be subjected to problem solving in the same manner as other problems. In some cases muscle tension and spasms may be relieved by muscle relaxation, dry mouth by sipping fluids regularly, dizziness by avoiding getting up quickly, restless legs by stretching exercises or physical exercise, increased appetite by careful dietary planning.

Patient and carer attitudes

Where patients and carers share constructive attitudes towards medication adherence to long-term regimens is likely to prove more successful. Patients or carers who are antagonistic towards drug taking readily sabotage compliance. Commonly expressed negative attitudes include:

'No drug should be taken for a long time. This leads to addiction, or at least to psychological dependence on the drug.'
'Drugs are for sick people only. But I'm not sick.'
'People who need drugs to stay well are weak characters. It is better to stay healthy through diet and exercise than through drugs.'

It is important to recognise that all these ideas have some validity and to acknowledge this with patients and carers. However, one or more educational sessions may be necessary to inform people of the benefits and unwanted effects of long-term drug therapy. The goal is to establish a network of informed consumers, who have sufficient knowledge to be able to participate constructively in monitoring all aspects of drug therapy. A balanced presentation of the nature of the medication that has been recommended, its mode of action, the problems likely to be encountered and ways of coping with them tends to help modify negative perceptions and to enhance compliance (McGill et al, 1983). At times anxiety about drug taking may have been conditioned by experiencing or witnessing severe drug reactions. A program of desensitisation and anxiety management may be needed to assist such people. Coercive attempts to establish drug taking may lead to increased fear and avoidance. Depot preparations that are given by intramuscular injection are a particular problem where persons are phobic of injections. Similarly, the need for plasma assays with lithium and other preparations may lead to reduced compliance in those persons with phobic reactions. The use of anxiety management strategies is frequently successful in overcoming these phobias which should be addressed with the same understanding as any other irrational fear responses.

The use of visual aids and handouts assists in the presentation of complex issues. We have developed a range of such materials for use in such education sessions on the drug management of schizophrenia, depression and manic disorders (see p. 202).

Maintenance of compliance

Once compliance has been established it should not be assumed that this will continue indefinitely. Persons who remain symptom-free for months may have little incentive for continuing to take medication. Missed doses are likely to become more frequent with time. Several strategies may be employed to avert this problem.

Taking medication to avert recurrences is not an inherently rewarding activity. External reinforcement that provides specific rewards for regular drug taking is one approach to supporting that behaviour. Once a behavioural pattern has been established it is not essential to provide reinforcement every time the behaviour is performed; intermittent reinforcement will suffice. Positive feelings expressed by carers at regular intervals is a simple method of reward. This may be accompanied by tangible rewards, such as a special meal, recreational outing, or small gift to express appreciation at less frequent intervals. One family allowed their daughter to choose a family outing once a month when she had taken more than 80% of her lithium tablets. This helped her maintain tablet taking, which formerly had become extremely irregular within months of recovery from a manic episode.

Praise and attention from the prescribing physician is cited by many patients as a valuable source of reinforcement for continued drug taking. Many perceived lack of such contact as signifying the relative insignificance of the treatment, particularly when their efforts to seek advice about side effects and other matters were not adequately addressed by other mental health professionals.

The advent of plasma level assays of many psychoactive drugs provides another avenue for positive feedback from physicians. Care should be taken that continued praise is given to patients who sustain therapeutic levels of drugs, and not merely to those who show subtherapeutic levels. A mutual interest in the levels and their association with compliance as well as other factors that may contribute to variation can be developed between patient and physician. A few patients metabolise drugs rapidly, and despite adequate compliance have undetectable or extremely low plasma levels. Such cases can be subjected to further testing. Doses can be given and serial plasma assays conducted at hourly intervals to ascertain the rate of metabolism. For such persons doses may have to be given more frequently, or alternatively, a depot preparation may be employed where available.

An added benefit from plasma assays is the ability to lower doses to the lowest possible level, confident that this should remain effective. There is a tendency in other circumstances to prescribe slightly more than needed in order to play safe. Such errors contribute to most persons receiving higher doses of drugs that they need with all the attendant problems of increased toxic effects and the desire to self-regulate to lower, often ineffective doses.

In summary, we have concluded that prophylactic drug therapy has proven highly effective in preventing recurrences of florid episodes of schizophrenic and major affective disorders. These benefits can only occur where effective adherence to long-term drug taking is maintained, usually for several years. This often entails a significant change in behaviour and attitudes, which cannot be taken for granted. We have employed a wide range of strategies to ensure that all persons receive the optimal amounts of drugs for their disorders at all times. This has resulted in minimal problems of poor compliance and has maximised the benefits of drug therapies.

Strategies for coping with persistent side effects

Whilst most side effects tend to improve with time, some persist and may even progress to major sources of impairment and disability. Indeed some effects of the drugs may be quite disabling, even when they are not experienced as irritants by the individual. For example, many neuroleptic drugs produce a staring quality in a person's facial expression. This facial expression may be interpreted as threatening by other people and have a profound effect on the ability to develop friendships. Thus, it is unwise to dismiss any subjective or objective unwanted effect as trivial, particularly where the drug is needed to be taken over an extended period.

We have already discussed many of the strategies employed to minimise these unwanted effects. Additional strategies include:

Monitoring side effects: a comprehensive check of side effects is conducted every three months. This includes the completion of a 35-item checklist, and a series of physiological and biochemical tests (see Figure 7.1). All mental health therapists are trained to conduct brief screening for tardive dyskinesia (based on Simpson et al, 1979), extrapyramidal symptoms, and cardiovascular abnormalities. Where the therapists detected any sign of serious side effects further examination was conducted by a psychiatrist.

Targeted drug taking: this method of targeting drug taking to those periods when the risk of recurrent episodes is high has been mentioned above. This is particularly useful for persons who are sensitive to drug effects regardless of dose or type of drug recommended. However, the principle of targeting all therapy to the optimal needed to maximise its benefit at any time supports the view that drugs should only be given when there is clear evidence that they are needed. With the possible exception of the membrane stabilising effects attributed to lithium salts, there is no clear evidence that any psychoactive drugs actually change the biological vulnerability to episodes of mental disorders. However, intermittent drug regimens can only be sustained where there is adequate teamwork between patients, carers and professionals. Furthermore, there is some evidence that rapid changes in drug dosage may increase the risk of side effects, so that gradual withdrawal and reinstatement of drug taking is recommended.

Stress management: the addition of psychosocial stress management appears to contribute to a reduced need for long-term drug prophylaxis (Vaughn & Leff, 1976), or at least allow reductions in the optimal doses required for protective effects (Falloon, 1985). These strategies will be described later in this chapter.

Most people are able to decide whether the discomfort of the drugs outweighs the benefits they confer in preventing recurrent episodes. It is crucial that the benefits as well as the unwanted effects of long-term drug regimens are reviewed on a regular basis. We ensure that this is done at least every three months. Patients and carers are integrated into this review process. Education about the drugs and their disorders is routinely provided so that they participate as informed consumers. They are encouraged to report any unusual

NAME _____ DATE _____

Drugs taken in the past week (and dosage):

A _____ B _____

C _____ D _____

Note the side effects experienced during the past week that have been attributed to each drug: A, B, C and D:

	Drug(s)	INTENSITY		
		Mild	Mod	Severe
1. Headache				
2. Dizziness/faintness				
3. Disturbed vision (eg blurred)				
4. Tinnitus				
5. Dry mouth				
6. Excess salivation				
7. Nasal stuffiness				
8. Breathing difficulties				
9. Rapid/irregular heart beat				
10. Nausea/vomiting				
11. Diarrhoea				
12. Constipation				
13. Appetite increase				
14. Appetite decrease				
15. Weight gain				
16. Excess thirst				
17. Taste abnormality				
18. Urination difficulty				
19. Menstrual problems				
20. Sexual dysfunction				
21. Muscle pains				
22. Muscle stiffness				
23. Slowed movements				
24. Muscle spasms				
25. Dyskinetic movements				
26. Tremor				
27. Skin irritation/rashes				
28. Tiredness/drowsiness				
29. Overactivity/elation				
30. Sleep disturbance				
31. Memory/concentration disturbance				
32. Confusion/disorientation				
33. Irritability				
34. Depressed mood				
35. Anxiety mood				

PHYSICAL FINDINGS

1. Weight _____
2. Pulse _____
3. BP _____
4. ECG _____
5. X-Ray _____
6. Haematol _____
7. Liver function _____
8. Renal function _____
9. Thyroid function _____
10. Biochem _____
11. Other: _____
_____
12. Drug levels _____
_____
_____

Figure 7.1. Buckingham side effects rating.

symptoms immediately so that measures to counter untoward effects can be initiated without delay and the benefits of drug prophylaxis can remain optimal throughout.

Education about mental disorders

One of the key developments in mental health care has been the education of sufferers and their carers about the nature of their disorders and the rationale for their clinical management. This development began in the early 1970s with Robert Liberman's educational seminars at the Oxnard Mental Health Center's model program in California (Liberman & Bryan, 1977). This work was further developed when it was found particularly helpful to family members, who had previously been left in the dark about the nature of the disorders from which their relatives suffered and the sorts of responses that they could make to assist in their recovery (Falloon et al, 1984, Chapter 5). Since that time numerous guides have been written and considerable efforts have been made to enhance consumer understanding of mental disorders.

The goals of education

The following goals have been set for the use of education in the prevention of recurrences of florid episodes of mental disorders:

(1) *To provide a rationale for treatment,* and thereby facilitate understanding about the need for long-term biological and psychosocial management for each patient and their carers.

(2) *To enhance self-management.* Patients and carers are encouraged to take an active role in the management of mental disorders. The index patient is considered to have particularly valuable understanding of the way in which his or her mental disorder contributes to his or her disabilities and handicaps, as well as the manner in which these limitations can be managed in everyday life. Education aims to support this 'expert' role, as well as the coping efforts of carers.

(3) *To develop a therapeutic alliance.* The therapist aims to establish him/herself as an honest, straightforward, supportive person, who is eager to learn from patients and carers as well as to share his or her professional 'secrets' as a key participant of the caring team.

(4) *To provide further assessment of patients and carers stress management skills.* Educational sessions provide the therapist with an opportunity to assess the manner in which care units have resolved major stresses in the past. Specific examples of their strengths and weaknesses of their problem-solving functions are noted.

We discuss in detail below the educational model that we have used in our integrated approach to the prevention of recurrent episodes, though the role of education and its use in various contexts is also described at various stages throughout this book.

Assessment of understanding of the index patient's mental disorder

We have devised a brief semi-structured interview that provides an assessment of the understanding of each person's mental disorder. This interview forms the initial part of a longer assessment that is employed for all people suffering from major mental disorders and their carers. The following topics are discussed with the index patient and each carer:

What do they understand about the disorder?
What is it called?
What do they think causes it?
What do they or others do that seems to make it better?
What do they or others do that seems to make it worse?
What are the benefits of current medications?
What are the undesirable effects of current medication?
What are the main personal difficulties that are associated with the disorder? Focus on specific examples.
What do they actually do to cope with these difficulties?
What other mental disorders run in the family? Are their other household members that suffer from stress-related health problems?

These interviews may be supplemented with standardised questionnaires that assess the factual knowledge of specific mental disorders. Examples of these are the Knowledge Questionnaire (KQ) (McGill et al, 1983) and the Knowledge About Schizophrenia Interview (KASI) (Barrowclough et al, 1987) which assess people's knowledge about schizophrenic disorders.

However, this assessment is focussed less on factual knowledge than on understanding of the vulnerability-stress model of mental disorders and its practical application in the reduction of impairment, disability and handicap associated with those disorders. For many this interview provides the opportunity to express their distress about their misfortune in suffering a major illness themselves, or in experiencing such a disorder in their intimate care network. The long-term threat associated with such an event might be expected to overwhelm the coping capacity of most people. Just as with other major life stresses such as bereavement or divorce, emotional responses may be poorly differentiated and hostility is sometimes directed towards the perceived source of the stress. Such emotional expression should not be considered a true reflection of the quality of ongoing relationships. The most extreme distress is associated with those with the poorest prognosis for short-term recovery. This poor outcome is most likely where these high levels of distress persist and seems to reflect excessive levels of life stress in the everyday life setting. We therefore view expression of this distress by carers as providing us with information about the levels of stress in the family resulting from a variety of reasons, rather than as indicators of particular personality characteristics or of poor overall coping ability.

Educational strategies

A wide range of strategies have been developed to educate patients and their carers about mental disorders and their clinical management. These have included reading materials such as pamphlets and books, video and audiotaped programmes, intensive one-day workshops, adult education courses, multi-family groups and home-based seminars. The relative merits of these various approaches have not been evaluated, but several critiques of the approaches have been published (Tarrier & Barrowclough, 1986; Cozolino & Goldstein, 1986).

The approaches we have employed have included most of these strategies, tailored to the specific needs of patients and carers. A set of written materials has been prepared on topics such as 'Coping with Depression', 'What is a Manic Episode?', 'Coping with a Manic Episode', 'What is Schizophrenia?' (also available on videotape), 'Treatment of Schizophrenia: Medication', 'Coping with Sleep

Disorders', 'Anxiety Management', 'Coping with Stress' (see pp. 222–223 for further details). In addition a small library of books and tapes has been acquired to lend to patients and carers.

It is not sufficient merely to acquire prepared informational materials and to distribute them to relevant persons in the hope that they will read the material and thereby acquire a comprehensive understanding of their disorders. Effective education must be targeted to the specific needs of each person. This includes consideration of the literacy skills, current information processing levels, as well as any substantial misunderstanding that may require special attention. Education is seen as a process that continues through all stages of the disorder, providing a constant frame of reference for all aspects of assessment and intervention. Furthermore, being a two-way process it enables the therapy team to acquire clearer understanding of the manner in which the disorder and its treatment affects the individual and his or her carers, as well as providing a rationale for clinical management. It is the key element in the integration of the person with the disorder and carers into the therapy team.

This is exemplified by the involvement of the index patient as a co-presenter of information about the disorder and its management to carers and professionals in educational sessions. Index patients are invited to share their first-hand experiences of their disorders and the effects of treatment strategies throughout the discussions. Carers are likewise invited to discuss the manner in which they have experienced the disorder and the impact of its management on their lives. Remarkably, for many this is the first time they have shared these experiences from their personal perspectives. This mutual disclosure within a supportive framework frequently results in dramatic enhancement of cohesiveness as people are able to make sense of abnormal behaviour patterns and to reattribute their origins to the effects of a disorder or its treatment. They may also be able to clarify factors that may have triggered episodes and to establish the earliest signs of a future episode. Relationships may be detected between changes in levels of impairment, disability and handicaps and biological changes, such as hormonal rhythms in women, levels of prescribed and non-prescribed drugs (including alcohol, nicotine and caffeine as well as illicit drugs), physical illness, and various environmental stressors. Such patterns provide support for the vulnerability-stress hypothesis, and, more crucially, clarify the rationale for the comprehensive biopsychosocial management of the disorder that aims to minimise all levels of morbidity on a long-term basis. It can be seen that education is the cornerstone of the approach we advocate.

In addition to the general approach outlined above, specific strategies used in education include:

Visual aids: Preparation of charts and diagrams that illustrate key aspects of the presentation of information is helpful. Care should be taken to ensure that the diagrams are clear and non-technical so that they clarify rather than confuse. Summaries of key points on a chalkboard, flash cards, flipchart or overhead projector may prove helpful.

Preparation for the presentation: Care should be taken to plan the educational session in detail. This necessitates reviewing the assessment of each participant's understanding; defining clear goals for each session, informing oneself of all important aspects, and choosing appropriate teaching aids, including pamphlets or books. Care should be taken to avoid technical jargon and to rehearse any aspects that the presenter may find difficult to present clearly.

Structuring sessions: Sessions are usually one hour long, but this may vary according to the information processing capacity of participants. With people who have a limited attention span it may be necessary to conduct educational sessions in 5–10 minute segments. This may be achieved by including an educational component as part of several sessions, or by breaking up the session into a number of segments interspersed by breaks of several minutes duration.

Maintaining attention: Ensuring that participants maintain attention throughout the session is important, even where deficits in information processing are absent. Information is best presented in blocks of not more than five minutes, with minimal interruptions. Participants are then invited to describe their own experiences, concerns or queries. It is often helpful to invite participants to summarise their understanding of the key points at the end of each issue that is discussed. This enables the presenter to identify areas where further clarification may be needed.

The involvement of the index patient as a co-presenter and resident 'expert' on his or her disorder helps maintain his or her attention throughout. Where that person is severely disabled it may be tempting to overlook his or her role and to conduct a dialogue about them between carers and professionals. It is crucial to avoid excluding the person in this manner. Requests for those who are disabled to assist in all aspects of the presentation, including the display of visual aids, and the clear reinforcement of this assistance by direct praise and gratitude for their efforts may support their continued involvement. It may be necessary to spend time with index patients before the session to prepare them for their role as co-presenters.

Control of emotional climate

The sessions are conducted in a calm, neutral manner, with the therapist avoiding taking sides or entering into debates on issues. Where a difference of opinion exists, this is clarified, without any coercion for people to change their views. Where clear-cut scientific evidence contradicts the opinion being expressed (e.g. persons with schizophrenia should never take neuroleptic drugs) the therapist restates the evidence to support the accepted opinion in a clear unequivocal manner. All constructive contributions by participants are acknowledged. *Hostile, accusatory or histrionic exchanges are halted immediately.* The therapist ensures that diversions from the key topics for the session are minimal.

Homework assignments

Participants are invited to study handouts and to identify any questions for further clarification or discussion at the beginning of the next session. Brief revision of the key points made at the previous session is made before reviewing the homework task at the beginning of the next session. Where substantial deficits in understanding remain further education may be needed, before moving on to other topics.

Continuing education

We regard education as a continual process. It is not sufficient to provide education at the start of treatment, and assume that people will remember all that has been said. This is particularly so if the education occurs when a participant's cognitive processes are impaired, either by a mental disorder, drug treatment, or the stress that they are experiencing. Revision and clarification of key aspects are addressed during all subsequent sessions. This may be particu-larly important at times of suboptimal compliance with any aspect of

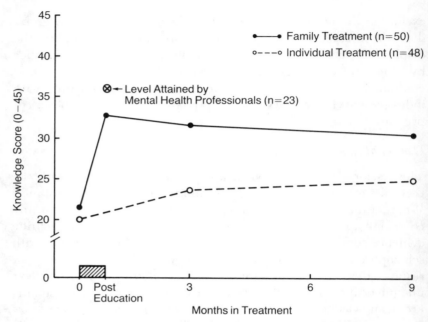

Figure 7.2. The acquisition and maintenance of knowledge about schizophrenic disorders after two educational sessions. (From McGill et al, 1983.)

the clinical management programme. Detailed assessments are made at 3-monthly intervals to ensure that relevant understanding is maintained at high levels. Although many educational programmes fail to enhance knowledge substantially, applying education in this manner has shown efficient, lasting acquisition of knowledge that has probably contributed to excellent engagement of persons in long-term prophylaxis with excellent compliance with the programmes (McGill et al, 1983; Figure 7.2).

Training people to monitor early warning signs

The outcome of most major mental disorders is better where episodes are treated optimally at the earliest possible time (Crow et al, 1986; Kupfer et al, 1989). The ability to recognise the earliest signs of an impending recurrence or exacerbation is a key element of effective long-term care. Training patients and their informal carers to recognise the earliest signs of such episodes and then to apply strategies to avert further deterioration with minimal delay may have major benefits.

The early signs of many disorders are remarkably similar. This should not be too surprising, as most represent the signs of excessive stress. Sleep and appetite disturbance, muscle tension pains, irritability and social avoidance are among the most common prodromal features of depressive (Fadden et al, 1987), schizophrenic (Herz & Melville, 1980) and anxiety episodes (Fava et al, 1988). The generic nature of these early signs might suggest that they would have very limited utility in defining the onset of episodes. This appears the case when they are aggregated into checklists (e.g. Birchwood et al, 1989). Fortunately, however, each persons tends to have a fairly specific pattern of signs that appear in a consistent fashion before a major episode. Furthermore, these signs do not appear at random. Rather they tend to be triggered by excessive life stress. This allows us to increase the sensitivity of our monitoring around periods of major stress, particularly those stressors that are not rapidly resolved and threaten to overwhelm the coping capacity of the person and his or her social support system.

We therefore include the monitoring of early warning signs as an extension of the education of all those who have experienced one or more episodes of a major mental disorder. Index patients and their carers attempt to recall the most striking features that preceded the onset of these episodes. When the episode has been very stressful it may be difficult to obtain clear recall. However, many relatives are extremely sensitive to these early signs and can identify idiosyncratic behaviour that precedes episodes in an uncanny way. The two or three specific features that provide the clearest indication of an impending episode for that particular individual are chosen. Care is taken to avoid features that may occur frequently in the absence of episodes. For example, George had experienced insomnia, appetite loss and headaches prior to his two schizophrenic episodes. However, he had headaches at least once a week, which although not as persistent, were identical in character. In contrast, his sleep and appetite were usually excellent. For this reason these last two features were chosen as his early warning signs.

Once the signs have been chosen the therapist attempts to define them as precisely as possible so that their emergence can be detected as clearly as possible, both by the index patient and carers. George's insomnia was defined as 'sleeping less than five hours a night, for two

---

EARLY WARNING SIGNS

Name: _JOY ALLEN_

I have a risk of developing episodes of a _SCHIZOPHRENIC_ disorder.

My early warning signs are:

1. _REDUCTION IN MY SLEEP OF 2 HOURS FOR 3 NIGHTS IN A ROW_

2. _NOT ABLE TO READ FOR MORE THAN 5 MINUTES AT A TIME_

3. _SPENDING MORE THAN 4 HOURS ALONE IN MY ROOM FOR 3 DAYS RUNNING_

Whenever I experience *any* of these signs I will respond by:

a) _INFORM MY DOCTOR BY PHONE IMMEDIATELY_

b) _INFORM MY THERAPIST (JAMES MCDOWELL) BY PHONE IMMEDIATELY_

c) _PINPOINT ANY STRESSES & ARRANGE EMERGENCY PROBLEM SOLVING DISCUSSION_

My Doctor is: _DR FRASER_ Phone: _819 468_

My Home Contact is: _JAMES MCDOWELL_ Phone: _829 641_

If I have any concerns about my disorder I will contact _JAMES McD_ immediately.

Figure 7.3. An example of an early warning signs card.

nights in a row'; and his appetite loss as 'eating less than half his evening meal on three consecutive nights'.

It is clear that the occurrence of such features may not always indicate an impending episode. However, they are employed as signals to the person and carers that vulnerability may be high, and that efforts to prevent an episode may need to be applied without delay. The response to early warning signs is individually contracted. In all instances the detection of signs leads to an emergency problem analysis by the therapy team. Patients and their carers are requested to contact the therapy team without delay. They are asked to err on the side of caution, and never to hesitate to call, even when they are not sure about the sign they have noticed. Telephone numbers are clearly noted on the Early Warning Signs forms that are displayed prominently in the home, as well as in the case records of both family practitioners and mental health therapists (see Figure 7.3). This problem analysis seeks to define the key triggers to the re-emergence of the disorder. These may be changes in vulnerability, stress, coping or biological buffers. Often the early warning signs result from a combination of several of these factors. For example, one young woman experienced early warning signs of a recurrence of manic episodes when she was in the premenstrual phase of her cycle, and had experienced a substantial increase in her ambient stress, when her highly supportive mother was abroad on holiday. In addition her medication had been discontinued. On rare occasions, no obvious precipitant of early warning signs can be identified, and it may be concluded that some endogenous factor, as yet not readily assessed may have been associated with the increased risk of a recurrent episode.

The therapeutic strategies employed to prevent the onset of a disabling episode of mental disorder after the prodrome has been detected include:

Education: Revision about the nature of the disorder and the principles that govern its effective clinical management.

Stress management: Problem solving to identify and resolve any current stressors. This includes not only any events or ambient stresses that may have triggered the prodrome, but also any persisting stresses that may be contributing to the overall stress impinging on the vulnerable person. This may include household stress that does not directly affect that person. For example, an argument between father and a brother had created considerable tension throughout one household that contributed to the stress experienced by his sister, who was recovering from schizophrenia.

Drug management: An increase in low-dose prophylactic drug therapy, or restarting intermittent drug therapy may be recommended.

Monitoring: The early warning signs are monitored on a daily basis to provide evidence of the effectiveness of the intervention program.

Reinforcement of detection process: It is crucial that the professional members of the community team reward the person and carers for making early contact whenever they suspect they have detected early warning signs. Often they may make contact when the signs are not precisely those defined as warnings, and often the signs will not be prodromes of any impending episode. However, it is crucial that all efforts to recognise signs and to provide an early assessment of potential episodes are clearly rewarded by the mental health team, including the family practitioner. Off-hand remarks may readily discourage people from subsequent efforts to seek advice at the earliest possible stage, and lead to consultation only when the episode has become fully established and in need of intensive care.

Follow-up: Further assessment and intervention may be provided to reduce the subsequent risk of recurrence. This may involve refinement of stress management or drug treatment procedures.

Training in stress management

The fourth component of our prevention of recurrence program involves enhancing the efficiency of management of environmental stresses by the index patient and his or her care unit. This is achieved mainly by increasing the efficacy of problem-solving strategies of the care unit.

Stress management is made up of five elements: (1) assessment; (2) education; (3) communication training; (4) problem-solving training; and (5) specific cognitive-behavioural strategies for specific problems. Evidence for its effectiveness in reducing recurrence rates in schizophrenia (Falloon, 1985) and affective disorders (Jacobson, 1988) is available from well-controlled clinical trials. The methods are detailed in Falloon et al (1984, 1988 & 1992). The main aspects of the approach will be summarised here.

Assessment

It should be recalled that all persons presenting to the service and their informal carers are assessed in terms of their capacity to manage all existing stresses in their lives, including the problem-solving efficiency of their family or household as a unit. When people present at the time of a major crisis this assessment may be focussed upon the current issues and may give a poor impression of problem-solving behaviour under less stressful circumstances. In any case, once the index patient's condition has stabilised a further review of the stress management skills of the care unit is undertaken. This may necessitate repeating the Individual Assessments of all household members, in addition to repeating the Problem-Solving Assessment. The focus of this review in terms of preventing recurrence includes the manner in which household members communicate about issues of personal and mutual concern, the nature of interpersonal support, particularly in assisting each other to achieve personal goals, the manner in which they resolve problems of everyday living, as well as major life crises, and the existence of any persisting stresses, including persisting impairments, disabilities and handicaps associated with the index person's mental disorder.

Education

The educational component of the program provides a clear rationale for adding stress management to optimal drug therapy in the prevention of recurrent episodes of most mental disorders. In addition to defining the early warning signs of impending episodes, patients and carers are invited to suggest major stressors that may have triggered past episodes. These may have been major life events or accumulated ambient stresses and burdens. For example, Sandra noted that each time she had experienced a manic episode her husband had been away on business overseas. This was not an unusual occurrence, but when he had been particularly stressed with special assignments in the weeks before a trip the household tension became high and this placed an extra burden on Sandra, especially in coping with their two teenagers. On such occasions her risk of recurrence was very high.

It is evident that clarifying links between stress and recurrence may lead to changes in peoples' lifestyles that result in improved management of stresses. However, mere insight into the association between certain stresses and episodes is insufficient to result in lasting beneficial changes and further intervention is necessary.

Communication training

The key goal of communication training is to enable people to express their needs and concerns in a clear direct manner to each other so that problem issues can be addressed in a straightforward manner. In other words, people living together in a household, or similar intimate network, can sit down together on a regular basis to discuss problems and personal goals in a supportive, constructive manner. Patients and carers are helped to express unpleasant feelings about problem issues in a way that facilitates problem solving and minimises interpersonal conflict. In addition, they are taught to listen empathically, to make requests in a constructive manner, and to express positive feelings for everyday pleasant events, including all efforts to resolve problems and achieve goals, regardless of the success that results from these efforts. These skills

Table 7.2. *Expressing unpleasant feelings*

LOOK AT THE PERSON: SPEAK FIRMLY
TELL THEM EXACTLY WHAT TRIGGERED YOUR UNPLEASANT
  FEELING
TELL THEM HOW YOU ARE FEELING
SUGGEST WAYS THAT THEY MIGHT HELP YOU GET RID OF THAT
  FEELING (Make a positive request or arrange problem-solving discussion)

---

are directed towards reducing ambient tensions of everyday life in the community as well as pinpointing major sources of stress that may require more elaborate problem-solving plans.

Communication training employs a skill-training approach with repeated practice of alternative strategies, with feedback, instructions, coaching, modelling and reinforcement of progress. Specific guidelines are provided for each communication skill (see Table 7.2). Considerable attention is devoted to ensuring that enhanced skills are incorporated into everyday social discourse. Homework assignments that promote daily practice with feedback are used to promote generalisation from treatment sessions to less structured interactions.

George had made repeated suicide attempts. Each episode had been triggered by some form of rejection in his work or social network. He tended to withdraw at these times despite efforts by his parents to discuss the issue with him. Assessment showed that he was unable to express feelings of frustration in a clear way to others. He was taught to express his feelings by stating exactly what he was frustrated about, how he felt about that situation, with appropriate non-verbal expression, and how he hoped the issue could be resolved. On the next occasion when he was stood up by a girl he had arranged to meet for a date, he returned home went to his room and locked the door. When his father went to ask him what was wrong he went to the door and told his father what had happened and how he felt devastated and wanted to kill himself. He agreed to sit down with his parents and discuss this issue. During the subsequent discussion he was able to resolve his concern that he would never establish a relationship with a girl, and begin to make plans for further forays into the treacherous waters of securing dates.

Problem solving training

Enhancing problem-solving skills is a strategy that has been discussed repeatedly in this volume. It is used by therapists as the basis for most aspects of their clinical management of all cases. The distinctive way in which it is applied in the prevention of recurrence is as a key strategy in stress management. Patients and carers are trained to use a structured problem-solving approach to provide clear plans for the achievement of their personal goals as well as to resolve problems. It is postulated that the efficient resolution of problems may contribute to effective stress management, so that even the most vulnerable persons may seldom exceed their stress thresholds and thereby risk experiencing a recurrence of their disorders. The accumulation of everyday hassles is considered as important as the advent of major life crises, so that emphasis is placed on using the problem-solving methods on a daily basis to deal with the whole range of stresses in the social network.

Although the six-step problem-solving approach is identical to that used in intensive crisis management, its use in a prophylactic context involves training the patients and carers to use the method themselves. The therapy sessions are merely workshops where the care unit learns to use the skills that they will subsequently employ in their own problem-solving discussions.

The six steps in this strategy are:

(1) *Problem definition:* The problem is pinpointed in a precise manner, so that all participants can collaborate in seeking possible solutions to a clearly defined issue. Often it is easier to provide a clear definition of a goal than a problem. A 'lack of friends' may become a goal of 'making a friend with one person of the same sex to go out with to a social event at least once a week'.

Of course, efficient problem or goal definition depends on effective communication skills, particularly active listening and clear expression of unpleasant feelings. The therapist prompts participants to employ these skills throughout the problem-solving discussion.

(2) *Brainstorming possible solutions*: The second step involves listing all possible solutions, regardless of their apparent effectiveness. At least five or six solutions are proposed and every suggestion is written down on the worksheet.

(3) *Evaluate each possible solution:* Each idea is then briefly discussed in terms of its possible benefits and disadvantages as a solution to that precise problem or goal. Benefits are always highlighted first.

(4) *Choose the 'best' solution:* There is seldom an ideal solution to any problem. This approach helps people to choose the solution that at this time best fits their needs and resources. This step may require some discussion, and again, effective communication skills will tend to facilitate this process.

(5) *Plan how to implement the solution:* A detailed step-by-step plan of action is established to ensure that the solution is implemented in the most efficient manner. Precise tasks are agreed, resources allocated, review procedures agreed, and plans made to cope with likely hitches. Difficult aspects of the plan may be rehearsed in role-played or real-life practice.

(6) *Review implementation:* A comprehensive review is conducted at a prearranged time. All efforts to carry out the plan are praised, regardless of how trivial, or more crucially, how successful. Further planning or problem solving is carried out where efforts have achieved limited progress towards resolving the problem or attaining the goal.

The same skill-training approach is used to train persons in the application of this problem-solving approach. Participants rehearse the skills during sessions with the therapist, who coaches them in the refinements of each component. In contrast to many therapeutic interventions, the therapist does not enter into the discussion, but provides guidance through constructive feedback, instructions, and where necessary by explicitly playing the role of one or more of the participants to demonstrate some aspect of the approach. The roles of chairperson and secretary are chosen from among the participants to facilitate efficient moving through each of the steps and keeping brief notes on the worksheets for future reference (see Figure 7.4).

The therapist aims to establish a regular (usually weekly) meeting between index patient and carers, where they convene their own discussions using this structured problem-solving approach. Once regular problem solving discussions have been established as part of the lifestyle in a household the therapist can withdraw into an advisory role, ready at all times to step in to assist with a major crisis or to assess any early warning signs of a possible recurrence. These weekly problem-solving discussions on matters of mutual concern to patients and carers are considered as important as regular drug-taking in the prevention of recurrence of major episodes. The same need to develop and then maintain adherence to this regimen is evident, all the more so because of the added complexity of requiring the compliance of several people.

Jackie and David were introduced to this aspect of relapse prevention after David had experienced a major depressive episode. They readily learned to carry out structured problem solving in the sessions convened by the

STEP 1: WHAT IS THE PROBLEM/GOAL?
Talk about the problem/goal. listen carefully, ask questions, get everybody's opinion. Then write down *exactly* what the problem/goal is.

Talk about the problem/goal. Listen carefully, ask questions, get everybody's opinion. Then write down *exactly* what the problem/goal is.

STEP 2: LIST ALL POSSIBLE SOLUTIONS.
Put down *all* ideas, even bad ones. Get everybody to come up with at least one possible solution. List the solutions *without discussion* at this stage.

1)

2)

3)

4)

5)

6)

STEP 3: DISCUSS EACH POSSIBLE SOLUTION.
Quickly go down the list of possible solutions and discuss the *main* advantages and disadvantages of each one.

STEP 4: CHOOSE THE "BEST" SOLUTION.
Choose the solution that can be carried out most easily to solve the problem.

STEP 5: PLAN HOW TO CARRY OUT THE BEST SOLUTION.
Resources needed. Major pitfalls to overcome. Practise difficult steps. Time for review.

Step 1)

Step 2)

Step 3)

Step 4)

STEP 6: REVIEW IMPLEMENTATION AND PRAISE *ALL* EFFORTS.
Focus on *achievement first. Review plan. Revise as necessary.*

Figure 7.4. A problem solving and goal achievement worksheet.

therapist. Jackie had a personal goal of finding a catering job nearer to home so that she would not have the stress of commuting some 50 miles. During one session they chose to work on plans for this goal.

Jackie defined the goal as finding a catering job near home. After some discussion they pinpointed this more exactly as:

To find a 9-to–5 job as a restaurant manager within 10 miles of home.

Possible solutions listed were:

approach all pubs and restaurants in the area
look for ads in papers

216 *Integrated mental health care*

speak to a friend in the business
go to job centre
give up work
start a family

It may be noted that some of the options do not appear to address the goal directly, and may be considered poor alternatives. However, these products of brainstorming often result in a focus on issues that are not considered in the usual convergent thinking employed in many of our problem-solving efforts.

The advantages and disadvantages of each of the solutions were highlighted and the couple decided that the best solution was to arrange a meeting with a friend who was very familiar with job opportunities available in the area. Having discussed this with her it was obvious that there was nothing available that would meet their requirements. On reviewing the issue David and Jackie decided that the most important thing was for Jackie to be able to spend more time at home at present, and that they would like to start a family. They therefore decided they would try to start a family in three months' time, once David had been fully rehabilitated in his work; and that Jackie would stop work after six months of pregnancy and find some part-time work close to home when she had stopped breast feeding.

This example is typical of many apparently straightforward problem issues that persons face. When a structured problem-solving method is used the issues are usually resolved quickly and without stress. It may be noted that this issue did not directly affect the index patient, and one might be tempted to conclude that this would have contributed little to preventing a recurrence of his depressive disorder. However, a stressed partner, who spends less time at home than she would like to, is less capable of providing additional support at times when this might be beneficial. Further-more, potential stressors for the relationship, such as the question of whether or when they might start a family, frequently surface within the supportive problem-solving context. It can be seen from this example that clear decisions can often be made with detailed planning. Although, these plans may not be realised precisely in the manner they had been laid out, the mere fact that the issue has been addressed in a direct, clear way tends to reduce the stress associated with uncertainty.

This problem-solving approach is remarkably similar to that employed in cognitive restructuring strategies that have been suc-cessfully developed for individual therapy with people with depres-sive and anxiety disorders (Beck et al, 1979; Beck et al, 1985). Although the cognitive therapy methods are a good deal more complex, and require extensive training, some researchers have suggested that similar results may be obtained with this much simpler problem-solving approach (Fennell, 1983). In our experience problem-solving methods have proven extremely useful in dealing with a wide variety of difficulties where stress plays a major role.

Specific cognitive-behavioural strategies

Many persons will experience persisting stress from a wide range of problems. These may include persisting disabilities and impairments from their disorders, including those associated with drug side effects, as well as lack of living skills in areas such as personal relationships, work and recreation. There may be occasions when patients and carers may find themselves unable to devise effective strategies to resolve these problems, which provoke a continuing source of stress. In such instances the therapist applies validated therapeutic strategies to supplement the problem solving. Strategies commonly applied are operant conditioning to enhance motivation to perform tasks that are not inherently rewarding, such as grooming and household chores, desensitisation procedures for specific anxiety, cognitive-behavioural strategies for depressive features, particularly the management of persisting low self-esteem and negative basic assumptions; social and leisure skills training for interpersonal problems and recreation; coping strategies for persistent hallucinations or delusions; and behavioural strategies for sexual dysfunction. These strategies may also be used to assist carers.

It is concluded that effective management of stress is a vital factor in the prevention of recurrence of mental disorders. A growing body of research suggests that these benefits are additional to those associated with drug prophylaxis, and can lead to a very low rate of recurrent episodes in schizophrenia and the major affective disorders (Lam, 1991). Stress management has benefits for carers as well, reducing their burdens and assisting in the achievement of their personal goals.

Casework strategies

The fifth component of the prevention of recurrence program is by
no means the least important. Although the model we employ
reduces somewhat the scope for traditional casework strategies such
as crisis intervention and counselling, it is crucial that expert
guidance is available to assist in resolving problems with finances,
benefits, housing, childcare, legal matters, education and work.
These problems contribute to persisting stress in a large proportion
of those who have experienced a mental disorder and it is crucial that
they are resolved efficiently. Casework is applied in a similar manner
to specific psychological strategies within the problem solving
framework. This ensures that patients and their carers are involved
as active participants in all aspects of the planning, and that they are
empowered to make full use of the resources and benefits that the
community provides.

Therapists do not do anything that the patients can do themselves. While it may seem easier for the therapist to make phone
enquiries to housing departments, or to provide information about
adult education programs, participants may gain much more from
seeking this information themselves and making personal contacts
with the relevant agencies. For example, Dawn was a single parent,
who was eager to join a mothers and toddlers group with her
daughter. She was anxious about how she would explain her
circumstances to anyone who asked about her husband. The therapist role-played this scenario with her so that she could try a number
of responses, until she felt confident that she could handle this issue.
Another example involved a couple who were eager to be rehoused.
They had been rebuffed on several previous occasions that they had
attempted to put their case to the local housing office. The therapist
problem-solved this issue with them, contributing her special knowledge of the way the office was managed. She suggested that they
insisted on meeting the chief housing officer and rehearsed with
them assertive responses to the receptionist's attempts to fob them
off. This plan resulted in the desired meeting with the officer and
while no apparent progress was made on the rehousing issue, they
felt that their understanding of the process involved was clarified
and considerable stress was removed.

Regular consultation with the specialist social worker is crucial to effective casework. This is provided through weekly team meetings, seminars and workshops on community resources and benefits, as well as guidebook references of local facilities. The close involvement of patients and carers in the teamwork enables them to provide details of local resources that are seldom known to the statutory agencies. Work, social and leisure opportunities are often found to fit the specific needs of particular disabled individuals, resulting in their comprehensive integration into the community. These issues are discussed in greater detail in the following chapter on rehabilitation.

Conclusion

It is concluded that recurrent episodes of mental disorders can be minimised by integrating biological and psychosocial strategies within the vulnerability-stress model. Optimal combinations of drug therapy, stress management and casework appear to reduce the risk of recurrences. Where episodes do recur, early detection at the prodromal stage ensures that intensive intervention is provided at the earliest possible stage. The need for highly efficient teamwork between all professions as well as with the index patients and informal carers is crucial to the success of this approach, as is the need to ensure that the key elements of the program are continually applied in an optimal fashion.

There is limited research to determine precisely how long this sort of program should continue after the last episode. Where persisting impairment and disability are evident it seems reasonable to assume that efforts to minimise this morbidity may need to continue indefinitely. However, in cases where a full remission is achieved the issue is unclear. The basic vulnerability to the disorder probably remains indefinitely, and may threaten to become manifest at any time. We have taken a two-year full remission of all impairment and disability as the minimum period for prevention of recurrence. After this time the program is gradually withdrawn. This usually begins with a gradual withdrawal from any prophylactic drugs, then a reduction of the frequency of psychosocial follow-up, particularly when it is evident that the care unit is conducting regular problem-solving discussions themselves and managing to cope with any ongoing stresses. Throughout this withdrawal phase careful monitoring of early warning signs is conducted. Patients and carers continue to monitor these indefinitely and contact their family doctors without delay when any signs arise. In addition, patients and carers are invited to contact the therapy team without hesitation at any future time that they feel they may benefit from professional assistance. The self-efficacy model that we employ ensures that such calls for assistance are made in a responsible manner, and seldom provoke any sense of burden on the professional resources.

References

Barrowclough C., Tarrier N., Watts S., Vaughn C., Bamrah J.S. & Freeman H.L. (1987) Assessing the functional value of relative's knowledge about schizophrenia. *British Journal of Psychiatry*, **151**, 1–8.

Beck A.T., Emery G. & Greenberg R. (1985) *Anxiety disorders and phobias: a cognitive perspective*. Basic Books, New York.

Beck A.T., Rush A.J., Shaw B.F. & Emery G. (1979) *Cognitive therapy of depression*. Guilford Press, New York.

Birchwood M., Smith J., MacMillan F., Hogg B., Prasad R., Harvey C. & Bering S. (1989) Predicting relapse in schizophrenia: the development and implementation of an early signs monitoring system using patients and families as observers, a preliminary investigation. *Psychological Medicine*, **19**, 649–656.

Brown G.W. & Harris T.O. (1978) *Social origins of depression: a study of psychiatric disorder in women*. Tavistock, London.

Cozolino L.J. & Goldstein M.J. (1986) Family education as a component of extended family-oriented treatment programs for schizophrenia. In M.J. Goldstein, I. Hand & K. Hahlweg (Eds.) *Treatment of schizophrenia*. Springer-Verlag, Berlin.

Crow T.J., MacMillan J.F., Johnson A.L. & Johnstone E.C. (1986) A randomised controlled trial of prophylactic neuroleptic treatment. *British Journal of Psychiatry*, **148**, 120–127.

Davis J.M., Schaffer C.B., Killian G.A., Kinard C. & Chan C. (1980) Important issues in the drug treatment of schizophrenia. *Schizophrenia Bulletin*, **6**, 70–87.

Fadden G.B., Kuipers L. & Bebbington P.E. (1987) Caring and its burdens: A study of the relatives of depressed patients. *British Journal of Psychiatry*, **151**, 660–667.

Falloon I.R.H. (1985) *Family management of schizophrenia*. Johns Hopkins University Press, Baltimore.

Falloon I.R.H. (1988) Expressed emotion: the current status. *Psychological Medicine*, **18**, 269–274.

Falloon I.R.H., Boyd J.L. & McGill C.W. (1984) *Family Care of schizophrenia*. Guilford Press, New York.

Falloon I.R.H., Laporta M., Fadden G. & Graham-Hole V. (1992) *Managing stress in families*. Routledge, London.

Falloon I.R.H., Mueser K., Gingerich S. et al. (1988) *Behavioural Family Therapy. A Workbook*. The Buckingham Mental Health Service, Buckingham.

Fava G.A., Grandi S. & Canestrari R. (1988) Prodromal symptoms in panic disorder with agoraphobia. *American Journal of Psychiatry*, **145**, 1564–1567.

Fennell M.J.V. (1983) Cognitive therapy of depression: the mechanism of change. *Behavioural Psychotherapy*, **11**, 97–108.

Ferris J. & Byer R. (1986) *Living with schizophrenia*. Newcastle-Upon-Tyne Polytechnic, Newcastle-Upon-Tyne.

Herz M. & Melville C.(1980) Relapse in schizophrenia. *American Journal of Psychiatry*, **137**, 801–805.

Jacobson N.S. (1988) Cognitive-behavioural marital therapy for depression. Paper presented at World Congress of Behaviour Therapy, Edinburgh, September 1988.

Kupfer D.J., Frank E. & Perel J.M. (1989) The advantage of early treatment intervention in recurrent depression. *Archives of General Psychiatry*, **46**, 771–775.

Lam D.H. (1991) Psychosocial family intervention in schizophrenia: a review of empirical studies. *Psychological Medicine*, **21**, 423–441.

Leff J. & Vaughn C. (1980) The interaction of life events and relatives' expressed emotion in schizophrenia and depressive neurosis. *British Journal of Psychiatry*, **136**, 146.

Liberman R.P. & Bryan E. (1977) Behavior therapy in a community mental health center. *American Journal of Psychiatry*, **134**, 401–406.

Mace N.L., Rabins P.V., Castleton B.A. et al. (1985) *The 36-hour day: Caring at home for confused elderly people*. Hodder & Stoughton, London.

Marks I.M. (1978) *Living with fear*. McGraw-Hill, New York.

McGill C.W., Falloon I.R.H., Boyd J.L. & Wood-Siverio C. (1983) Family educational intervention in the treatment of schizophrenia. *Hospital and Community Psychiatry*, **34**, 934–938.

Parkes C.M., Brown G.W. & Monck E.M. (1962) The general practitioner and the schizophrenic patient. *British Medical Journal*, **ii**, 872.

Paykel E.S. (1978) Contribution of life events to causation of psychiatric illness. *Psychological Medicine*, **8**, 245–253.

Prien R.F. (1984) Long-term maintenance pharmacotherapy in recurrent and chronic affective disorders. In M. Mirabi (Ed.) *The chronically mentally ill: research and services*. New York, Spectrum.

Rowe D. (1983) *Depression: The way out of your prison*. Routledge & Kegan Paul, London.

Schou M. (1989) Lithium prophylaxis: myths and realities. *American Journal of Psychiatry*, **146**, 573–576.

Seeman M.V., Littman S.K., Plummer E., Thornton J.F. & Jeffries J.J.
    (1982) *Living and working with schizophrenia.* University of Toronto
    Press, Toronto.
Simpson G.M., Lee J.H., Zoubak B. & Gardos G. (1979) Rating scale for
    tardive dyskinesia. *Psychopharmacology,* **64,** 171–179.
Soskis D.A. (1978) Schizophrenic and medical inpatients as informed
    drug consumers. *Archives of General Psychiatry,* **31,** 645–647.
Tarrier N. & Barrowclough C. (1986) Providing information to relatives
    about schizophrenia: some comments. *British Journal of Psychiatry,*
    149, 458–463.
Vaughn C.E. & Leff J.P. (1976) The influence of family and social
    factors on the course of psychiatric illness. A comparison of
    schizophrenic and depressed neurotic patients. *British Journal of
    Psychiatry,* **129,** 125–137.
Wing J.K., Bennett D.H. & Denham J (1964) The industrial
    rehabilitation of long-stay schizophrenia patients. *Medical Research
    Council Memo* No.42, H.M.S.O., London.

Bibliography of educational materials

Anxiety disorders

Marks I.M. (1978) *Living with fear.* New York, McGraw Hill.
Butler G. (1985) *Managing anxiety.* Oxford, University of Oxford.

Depressive disorders

Falloon I.R.H. (1985) *Coping with depression.* Buckingham, England:
    Buckingham Mental Health Service.
Rowe D. (1983) *Depression: The way out of your prison,* London: Routledge
    & Kegan Paul.

Schizophrenic disorders

Birchwood M. & Smith J. (1985) *Understanding schizophrenia.* Birmingham,
    England: West Birmingham Health Authority Mental Health
    Series.
Seeman M.V., Littman S.K., Plummer E., Thornton J.F. & Jeffries J.J.
    (1982) *Living and working with schizophrenia.* Toronto: University of
    Toronto Press.
Falloon I.R.H., McGill C.W. & Boyd J.L. (1980). *What is schizophrenia?*
    and *Treatment of schizophrenia: Medication.* Los Angeles: University of
    Southern California. (Videotape also available.)

Manic disorders

Hole V. & Falloon I.R.H. (1987) *What is a manic episode?* and *Coping with a manic episode.*, Buckingham, England: Buckingham Mental Health Service.

Childhood behaviour disorders

Patterson G.R. (1971) *Families*. Champaign, Illinois: Research Press.

Dementing disorders

Mace N.L., Rabins P.V., Castleton B.A. et al (1985) *The 36-hour day: Caring at home for confused elderly people*. London: Hodder & Stoughton.

8

Integrated clinical management of the long-term disabled

One of the greatest challenges faced by any mental health service is how to ensure that people with disability and handicaps associated with mental disorders receive effective management until their psychosocial morbidity has been minimised and they are participating in all aspects of life they choose to in the community (see Table 8.1). It is not considered sufficient merely to eliminate the impairment (psychopathology) of the mental disorders. Effective clinical management aims to restore functioning so that people can resume life of a similar quality to the one they would have enjoyed if they had not suffered the misfortune of developing a mental disorder. Once restored, it is crucial to ensure that such effective functioning is maintained. Thus, the aim of the integrated approach is to restore and maintain comprehensive functioning in the community.

This rehabilitative approach is applied to every case and every carer from the onset of clinical management and continues until all residual morbidity has been eliminated. For some people this may occur within weeks or months, for others therapeutic strategies must be maintained indefinitely in an attempt to restore functioning. Present clinical management is not capable of facilitating complete functional recovery in every case. However, this should not deter services from continual efforts to assist disabled people to maximise their creative potential within the constraints imposed upon them by their disorders. In contrast with many hospital-based services, the integrated approach does not accept that life out of hospital and prevention of readmission as a sufficient goal. We believe that it is the quality of life of patients and their carers that is the ultimate measure of an effective service to a community. This chapter will describe the strategies that we employ in the resolution of long-term

224

Table 8.1. *Impairment, disability and handicap*

Impairments	Disabilities	Handicaps
Thought interference	Cognitive:	Lack of friends
Perceptual distortion	inefficient problem solving,	Unemployment
Motor abnormality	slowed learning	Limited leisure
Reduced attention	Affective:	activity
span	inappropriate fear, feelings of	Poor housing and
Reduced drive	inadequacy	self-care
Impaired function	Behavioural:	Carers burdened
	low rate of constructive actions	

management of disability and handicap associated with mental disorders.

In order to meet the needs of people with disability and handicap associated with mental disorders an effective service needs:

1 Clear goals to allocate service resources according to the level of disability of patients and their carers.
2 Procedures to implement cost-effective intervention strategies that address all the specific biopsychosocial needs of all disabled individuals.
3 A case management system that ensures that continuous monitoring of personal goals, impairment, disability and handicap enables treatment strategies to be adapted to the changing needs and problems each person encounters.
4 An identical process of case management for key carers, to ensure that their personal goals are being achieved, and impairment, disability and handicap minimised.

As mentioned in earlier chapters, one of the central goals of an integrated community service is that priority is given to those with mental health disorders where the risk of long-term disability and handicap is greatest (i.e. mainly schizophrenic, major affective, and major anxiety disorders). The vulnerability to developing major impairment associated with these disorders is frequently long term and severe disabilities and handicaps are common. The principle guiding our work is that people with disabling forms of these disorders and their carers receive continuous treatment while clinical and social morbidity or major stress and vulnerability factors remain evident. Moreover, they are systematically monitored until they have been free of symptoms or disability for a further period of

two years. Some people continue to be monitored after this time i
there is concern that they may have a history suggesting a high risk o
recurring episodes of serious impairment or disability. In practic
this means that some people are monitored by the mental healt
services all the time, as they never experience a period of two year
when they are fully functioning and impairment-free.

Those whom we define as being in need of long-term cas
management meet one of the following criteria:

1 Anyone with a major mental disorder (Axis 1, DSM III-R
needing clinical management (including relapse prevention) fo
one year or longer.
2 Anyone who registers with a family practice in the area who ha
had a major mental disorder for which they have needed clinica
management during the previous year.
3 Anyone having an episode characterised by clear prodroma
features of a schizophrenic or major affective disorder.
4 Anyone who has clearly recognised vulnerability factors tha
suggest they have a high risk of developing serious disability fron
a mental disorder in the future.

When people are first referred to an integrated service, thei
names are entered on a database, and therapists can therefore b
easily alerted to the fact that they should enter the long-term
management programme if they are still in treatment after one yea
has elapsed since referral. Therapists regularly monitor their owr
caseloads, at least every three months, to identify people who hav
become 'long-term' during the previous three months. Family prac
titioners and their clerical associates are reminded to alert thei
teams if anyone who has a current or past history of a menta
disorder registers with them so that the situation can be assesse
and appropriate clinical management begun immediately. This i
especially important for people who have moved to the area recently
The stresses involved in relocation are often sufficient to provok
recurrences even in people who have achieved stable long-term
remissions.

Assessment

When a person enters the long-term care program a detailed an
comprehensive review of their current impairments, disabilities an

handicaps is conducted. Vulnerability, stress and coping capacity is reviewed along with progress towards resolution of targeted problems and achievement of personal goals. A similar review is carried out with key carers. Decisions about any modification in the clinical management plans are always based on this thorough assessment. The emphasis on this comprehensive assessment is derived from a goal of working towards maintaining and restoring optimal functioning rather than simply being interested in improvement in symptomatology. Assessments are carried out even where there are no apparent difficulties, as there are almost always areas in which further improvements in functioning and quality of life can be achieved with additional therapeutic input from the multidisciplinary team. It is also important to be aware in advance of any anticipated life events or crises which may contribute to relapse or a lessening of the person's or family's ability to cope. It is important to work on vulnerability factors and to help people to improve their problem-solving skills, their social and interpersonal living skills, and work/activity skills so that their ability to cope is enhanced.

Assessment covers the following areas:

Review background history of disorder: Previous episodes; response to past clinical management, best levels of psychosocial functioning – social, interpersonal, educational, occupational, leisure and recreational, intimacy, childrearing, etc. Social disadvantages – social deprivation, cultural factors.

Impairment: Detailed description of persisting psychopathology in terms of severity, frequency of *targeted symptoms*; as well as recent evidence of *early warning signs*. Review impairment associated with drug treatment including side effects (see Figure 8.1).

Disability: Assessment of disturbance of psychological functioning associated with impairment – cognitive processing, emotional responses, behavioural performance in pursuit of everyday living goals; strategies used to cope (problem solving skills) with functional impairments and current and impending stresses; understanding of the nature of the disorder and treatment; compliance strategies. Each person's repertoire of living skills is reviewed. These include:

personal care skills
independent living skills
conversational skills

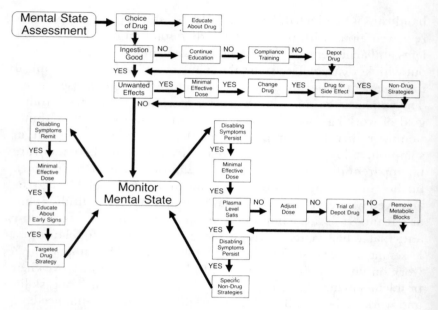

Figure 8.1. A flowchart for targeting long-term drug intervention strategies.

vocational skills
recreational skills
friendship and intimacy skills
self-help skills
problem-solving skills
stress management skills

Handicap: Assessment of social disadvantages that prevent achievement of everyday personal goals – carer support, social network support, availability of potential friends, work, leisure and recreation, housing, finance and transport.

Several standardised questionnaires have been developed to aid the therapist in assessing all relevant living skills and community needs (Baker & Hall, 1983; Wallace, 1990). This assessment process is summarised in Figures 8.1–8.4.

Following this general assessment of a patient it often becomes clearer which areas he or she experiences minimal difficulties and those areas that may need more detailed assessment. Decisions are then made about where our interventions should be targeted. Any of

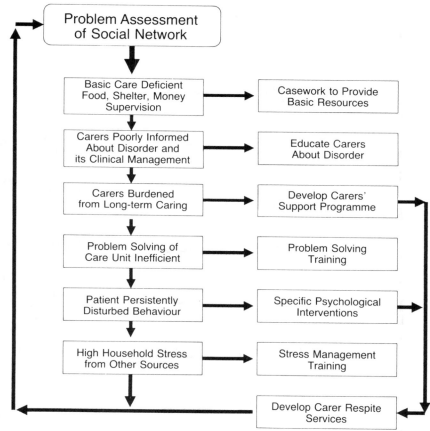

Figure 8.2. A flowchart for targeting support network intervention strategies.

the areas mentioned can become the focus of intervention, and therapy is provided by one or more members of the professional team as appropriate.

The order in which problem areas are prioritised for intervention is usually based on the following considerations:

1 Difficulties which patients and carers identify as the most important for them to tackle first. These are frequently problems which are currently interfering with a person's ability to cope or are threatening to overwhelm their coping capacities and cause persistent disability.

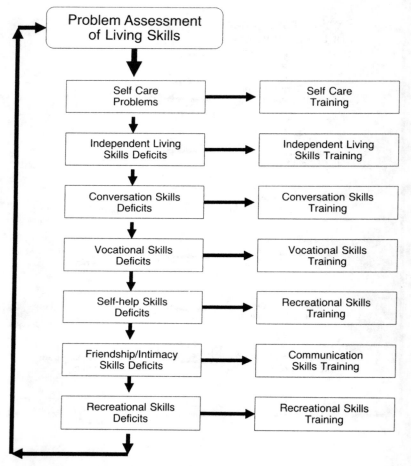

Figure 8.3. A flowchart for targeting living skills training strategies.

2 Basic skills that must be acquired as a prerequisite for learning
   more sophisticated skills, e.g. basic self-care skills such as grooming must be present before advancing to friendship and intimacy
   skills, and interview skills may need to be improved before a
   person may be successful in acquiring a job.
3 Difficulties that are likely to interfere with attempts to deal with
   other problems. Examples include poor compliance with medication, lack of understanding of the disorder on the part of the

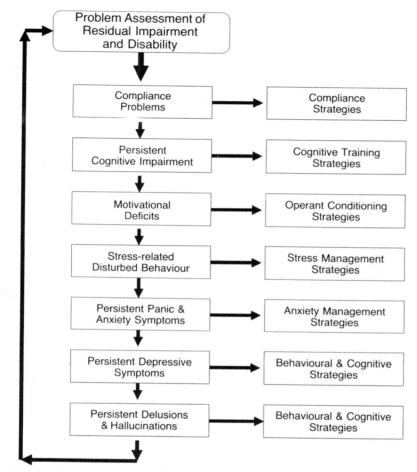

Figure 8.4. A flowchart for targeting specific psychological interventions.

patient or carers, persistent hallucinations or delusions, and problems with housing or finance.

The clinical management plan is always negotiated with patients and carers as part of their problem-solving sessions. At no stage does the therapist impose any therapeutic strategy that the care unit (patient and carers) can undertake themselves in a competent manner. This may include seeking assistance of community agencies, skills training, or finding out details about community resources. The therapist provides guidance and reinforcement for their efforts and specific therapeutic strategies that are not in the everyday repertoire of the care unit. This approach validates the efforts of the patient and carers and tends to enhance their willingness to work on the difficulties they consider most relevant while increasing the capacity of the professional service to provide that assistance that cannot be provided through existing informal resources. This is a further example of the way the service integrates with effective community efforts, rather than replacing these resources with professional assistance of doubtful superiority. Of course where skills and resources are inadequate, or people are overburdened by their efforts, the mental health professionals may provide more extensive input, at least for short periods, and in a targeted manner.

Intervention strategies

There are relatively few replicated controlled research studies that specifically examine the effectiveness of rehabilitation strategies. Most studies of long-term clinical management have focussed on the prevention of recurrent episodes, rather than improving the quality of life of sufferers and carers. However, a few studies have addressed both these issues, and offer guidance on the cost-effectiveness of specific approaches. A series of drug studies has demonstrated that psychosocial functioning can be enhanced for people who are recovering from schizophrenia when oral preparations are carefully monitored (Falloon et al, 1978; Schooler et al, 1980; Hogarty et al, 1979), or when low dosage strategies are employed with depot administration (Kane et al, 1986; Carpenter et al, 1987; Marder et al, 1988). Skills training methods have been effective in reducing disability in schizophrenia (Wallace & Liberman, 1985) and in depressive disorders (Bellack et al, 1983). Carer-based management that employed a mixture of education, problem solving, interpersonal skills training and specific cognitive-behavioural strategies has proven effective in reducing disability in schizophrenia (Falloon, 1985). A similar combination of behavioural strategies was effective in the rehousing of long-term mental hospital residents into community settings (Paul & Lentz, 1977). This latter project employed operant strategies to prompt and reward appropriate social behaviour patterns. Both these comprehensive behavioural approaches demonstrated superior cost-effectiveness to the less structured traditional approaches to rehabilitation. Furthermore, the approach was targeted to the specific needs and personal goals of every individual.

The amount and type of intervention provided to each individual or care unit obviously depends on the nature of the deficits and goals to be addressed. However, most effective intervention strategies have a common emphasis on education and understanding of the rationale for this approach; active involvement of carers and other relevant people in the person's social network; the setting of specific achievable goals; a structured skills training approach; review of effects following implementation of the treatment plan, and continuous amendment or reformulation of plans until the desired goals are achieved. Many aspects of these assessment and intervention approaches have been described in depth in other chapters. Particular issues arise, however, when working with people with long-term disability and handicap.

Education

It is often assumed when someone has experienced several episodes of a disorder that they and their carers understand all aspects of the disorder and its management, particularly if they have had the good fortune to discuss the disorder with a mental health specialist. However, this is often not the case, and even when people take part in educational sessions as described in other chapters, information is frequently not retained. Several factors can contribute to this:

People forget what they have been told especially if they are dealing with unfamiliar topics.

Information that is necessary is retained, and that which is not is used frequently is not. If people experience infrequent episodes of a disorder, they sometimes do not retain the information they were at one time familiar with.

Dealing with the stress of long-term disorders is difficult, and when under pressure, people do not always retain information or can find if difficult to gain access to the information they already have.

Gaining an understanding of mental disorders can be a complex task. People very often retain their own views about what is wrong and spend time testing out the validity of information provided by professionals before accepting it.

Children's ability to understand changes as they develop. Their understanding of a parent's disorder therefore may not be accurate if it has been some time since their parent experienced an episode of the disorder.

Many mental disorders impair the person's ability to concentrate and retain information at different points in time.

For these reasons it is essential when dealing with long-term disorders to provide ongoing opportunities to check patients' and carers' understanding of the disorder. Any information provided should be clear and reviewed frequently. It is helpful to leave reading material that people can re-read at their own pace.

Therapists working with people over long periods of time can very often become unaware of the need to go over information many times, feeling that they have covered the topic already. In situations like this we have found that it is useful for a therapist to have co-workers. When one therapist is involved with people less frequently, they often notice things which somebody in very regular contact misses.

John was a 45-year-old man who lived with his wife and two children aged 12 and 8. He experienced recurrent episodes of paranoid psychosis which resulted in great disruption to his lifestyle and that of his family.

In spite of continued family-based case management, they lacked an ability to detect the early warning signs of impending deterioration in John's disorder, or to note a reduction in his compliance with medication. This was accompanied by a reluctance to inform the mental health team that the situation was becoming difficult to cope with.

The team, therefore, continued to focus attention on education about the disorder and about the value of continued low-dose medication which appeared to produce rapid improvement in John's impairment and associated cognitive deficits. After several mild exacerbations, John and his wife began to recognise his early warning signs, to make sure that he took his medication regularly at those times, and to target problem solving to any stressors that may have triggered the exacerbation. This enabled him to spend less time off work and to put more effort into a home improvement project that was one of his personal goals.

It is also especially important when people move to the area with a pre-existing disorder that a careful assessment is made of their understanding of what is wrong, and what they have been told in the

Table 8.2. *Living skills training assessment*

Set personal goals
What skills are needed to achieve goals?
Deficits in receiving and information processing skills?
Deficits in repertoire of relevant skills?
Deficits in real-life performance of skills?
Adequacy of self-reinforcement for competent performance of skills?
Reinforcement from carers and social network?
Accessibility of community resources for disabled without
discrimination?

past. Very often people have received inaccurate or inadequate information, and this situation must be remedied as soon as possible. In addition, the relapse prevention strategies, including optimal drug prophylaxis and carer-based stress management need to be initiated at an appropriate time, along with efforts to overcome any residual disability or impairment.

Training in community living skills

Successful community living requires an extensive repertoire of skills, ranging from basic self-care, work and leisure, to interpersonal and intimacy skills (see Figure 8.3). A lack of effective skill performance in any key area may handicap any person from achieving the goals that they aspire to. A wide range of deficits may contribute to a lack of competent skill performance. The major areas are summarised in Table 8.2. In order to improve a person's living skills these components need to be assessed and strategies devised to correct major deficits or to cope with persisting disabilities. Thus, assessment must determine whether a person is able to receive and process social cues in an accurate and appropriate manner so that his choice of response to a specific situation will be optimal; the individual's repertoire of skills in the area of concern must provide an adequate range of appropriate responses; he or she must have the confidence to perform those skills; and finally, the individual must assess the effectiveness of their own performance in a constructive manner, with self-reinforcement for efforts, and encouragement from carers and friends in his or her social network. All skill training methods provide repeated real-life practice of skills as the basis for training (see Figure 8.5). In addition, it may be necessary to add specific

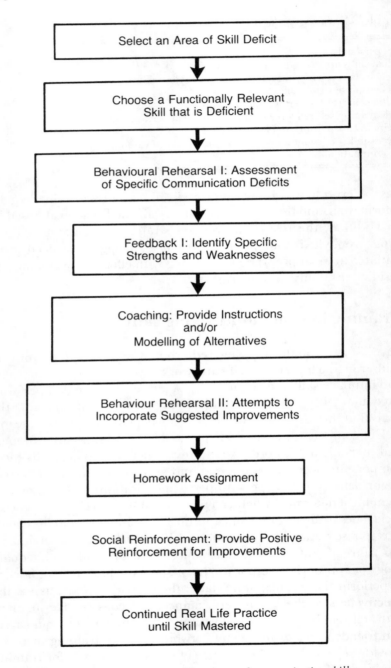

Figure 8.5. Assessment and training of interpersonal communication skills.

cognitive training to enhance reception of social cues and accurate information processing, anxiety management, cognitive strategies to enhance self-esteem and accurate constructive self-appraisal, and enhanced carer and peer support for efforts rather than achievements (Liberman et al, 1989).

Because all long-term cases in the integrated service receive training in communication and problem-solving skills with their carers as part of their relapse prevention, they have already learned to use the skill training model. Thus, subsequent intervention is conducted within the carer/family problem-solving and goal achievement framework. Skills which any household member wishes to develop in order to achieve their personal goals may be addressed in these sessions. Where these involve issues outside the household, the other participants may assist with role-played practice, and subsequently prompt and reward real-life performance. On occasions the therapist may undertake to accompany the patient on a real-life assignment, such as a job enquiry or interview, to a community activity, or to practice shopping at a supermarket. At all times the therapist performs the role of a coach, rather than a friend, prompting *in vivo* rehearsal of skills, and providing feedback and reinforcement of performance. Naturally the therapist behaves in a warm and friendly manner, but their role is clearly acknowledged as that of a professional engaged in rehabilitation training.

The advantages of providing skills training in peoples' own homes and in the villages and places where they live, work and play are obvious. It is possible to get a very accurate and detailed picture of where someone lives, what facilities they have at hand, situations that cause difficulty, and problems that are encountered. Therapists can actually experience for themselves the settings in which people live – can understand how difficult it is for Jackie to find space for herself in her two-bedroomed house; can hear for themselves the noise coming through the thin walls from next door which Dave has to endure when trying to relax; can realise why Joan thinks it is too big a step to go on her own to the local bus-stop having walked it with her; can be aware of the size and lay-out of the supermarket where Sandra hopes to be able to do her shopping; can appreciate John's concern that the neighbours are watching him, having been able to observe the neighbours' activities while standing with John in his living room. This experience and information is invaluable for therapists in helping them to assist in planning the most appropriate interventions in each situation. It also reduces the likelihood of misinterpreting statements and ideas which may sound odd or bizarre when in fact they are true. It makes it less likely that relevant facts are forgotten, which is often the case when simply asking people about situations. It also means that the problems of transfer of skills from one situation to another are lessened thus avoiding replication of input and ensuring that people can apply skills where they need to as quickly as possible. Finally, it facilitates stress management, so that people can plan their daily activities to maximise progress towards their personal goals without exceeding their thresholds of vulnerability where stress exceeds their capacity to cope, and may interact with their biomedical status to produce further risk of major episodes of impairment.

Community resources

As therapists develop greater knowledge of the social habitats of patients and their carers, they become increasingly aware of the myriad of resources that even deprived communities can provide for disabled people. Compared with the best equipped occupational and recreation therapy units in mental hospitals, the community offers a much broader range of opportunities and facilities. In common with most of us, people who are recovering from mental disorders are often unaware of the resources in their neighbourhoods, and complain that they can find no leisure or work activity to meet their special requirements. Reports such as this, taken at face value, lead to mental health services planning special activity centres, sheltered work programs and special day care units, to replicate those found in the large institutions. Not surprisingly these units are used no more than they would be if attendance at their equivalent programs in the hospital was made optional and nurses did not ensure that patients got up, showered, dressed and went off to the various units every morning. Indeed, Richard Lamb (1979) noted that attendance at such centres in the community tended to fall off dramatically when the centre was not within a short walk or easy bus journey from the person's home.

The disabilities associated with mental disorders that place constraints on people's community functioning are mainly those associated with a reduction in cognitive capacity, that interferes with attention and concentration, and slows thought and decision making processes. While this may limit a person's capability to return rapidly to jobs that depend on a high cognitive capacity, or to tackle goals that may create excessive stress, there are very few who will not be able to find a wide range of suitable leisure and recreational activities in their neighbourhoods. The greatest problem will be ability to seek and gain access to such resources. Apart from the planning needed to seek out these resources, to acquire adequate finances to pay any fees, and to travel to the resources, the greatest hurdle is probably the manner in which many people in the community still discriminate against people who have had mental disorders. A crucial role for mental health therapists in an integrated service is to break down this segregation and the unfounded anxiety that many members of the community have about the behaviour of people disabled from mental disorders. As with any anxiety, no amount of rational discussion is as effective as real-life exposure to the feared object. Thus, encouraging patients to access community resources and show people that they are ordinary responsible citizens, not violent, unpredictable, or irresponsible individuals, is probably the most efficient way of gaining greater acceptance and support for the disabled. The development of special units that segregate the mentally disordered, serves to perpetuate fears that these people cannot be integrated into everyday community activities.

Once again, where the integrated problem-solving efforts of the mental health therapists with the patient and carers fails to develop an effective plan to deal with a particular goal or problem, the service may support those people with a referral to a specialised unit, such as a sheltered workshop, training centre, day centre or residential rehabilitation unit that provides exclusively for the needs of people recovering from mental disorders. We have found the needs for such specialised resources minimal, and that the disadvantages of grouping together people with a wide range of needs and goals tend to outweigh the potential benefits of such special programs. Of course working in this way is more difficult for therapists than merely making referrals to a few specialised units then blaming the patients for non-attendance. Without ready-made solutions, finding and planning the resources that match individual needs can take weeks or months. However, throughout that time, patients and carers are actively engaged in a learning exercise, and may use their time to further build the skills they will need in order to succeed with their goals without experiencing excessive stress.

The following is an example of the way in which community resources are accessed in an integrated community service:

Simon: a 20-year-old who had dropped out of university. His family attempted to help him develop leisure activities that would enable him to achieve his personal goal of having a close male friend who he could chat with on a regular basis. The early problem-solving efforts centred around plans to renew contact with old school friends who still lived locally. This plan was a partial success, but did not result in any lasting friendship. Simon, his family and therapist agreed that it might be worth taking a different tack, and finding a regular leisure pursuit where Simon would meet a wider range of potential friends, all with some common interest. In a problem-solving session with the therapist they brainstormed all the possible activities and places that were available in the community that might be worth considering. These included:

going to the library to find a list of clubs
local football club
local pub darts team
night classes in computers, or photography
season ticket at football club
singles clubs
bus excursions
church groups
music groups, choirs, etc.
ramblers
Rotaract, young adults community action groups
historical society
swimming
badminton club
volunteer work
basketball club
jazz evenings
political groups
archeological digs
share a house with other young people
go to community events
join friendship circle (co-sponsored by a charity and mental health service
    – therapists' suggestion)

Over six weeks Simon sought further information about a selection of these ideas and tested out several. He worked on improving his conversational skills during weekly sessions with the therapist and his mother, father and 18-year-old brother. At the end of this period he had joined the local church choir, joined a conservation group who were working on a project to restore an historic site, and had begun to develop a friendship with a young man who shared both these interests. He was still working on developing a sporting activity and was expressing concern that he was gaining weight and not keeping fit. He had spent a free evening in a new health club, but realised that he could not afford the fees.

Work activity and vocational skills training

Work is a vital component of life in industrialised countries. Traditionally, this included work in the home, including childrearing and health care for women and work outside the home for men. Recent trends have led to a breakdown of many of these traditional roles, with women and men sharing work activities inside and outside the home. However, vocational rehabilitation in mental health has been slow to adjust to these trends and most programs offer a narrow range of training that is seldom geared to job opportunities in the local community.

While there is no doubt that work that is rewarded with sufficient pay to enable a person to support themselves and others is highly valued in our communities, the stresses this often entails may prove detrimental to many people with persisting disability associated with mental disorders who may gain considerable satisfaction from adapting to less stressful non-remunerative work in the community (Wing et al, 1964). A recent study of disabled people in the US showed that the unemployment rate was 80% (Goldstrom & Manderscheid, 1982). Although this data undoubtedly reflects the ineffectiveness of most mental health services to restore job functioning for many cases, it may also suggest a narrow approach to work activity that devalues alternatives to paid employment outside the home. The integrated community approach always starts with the personal goals of the patients and carers. For many people, their goal is clearly that of early return to a highly valued job. For others the opportunity, at least for a brief period, to explore constructive alternatives, may be welcomed. For example:

Jack, was a 34-year-old man, who had worked as a long-distance truck driver for many years, was delighted with the opportunity to spend more time at home with his two children. He took over much of the home management from his wife while she returned to work as a schoolteacher. He decided not to go back to trucking as he realised the stresses of constantly being on the road and having to meet deadlines were too much for him. He bought a new car and joined the local taxi service, a job where he could work flexible hours that fitted into home-life, and provoked minimal stress.

Work skills vary substantially from job to job. Among those common to most jobs are:

    job seeking
    job application and interviews
    travel to job and punctuality
    personal appearance and hygiene
    conversational skills
    problem-solving skills
    planning daily activity schedule
    active listening to instructions
    handling criticism
    pacing one's efforts
    tolerating routine, repetitive tasks
    stress management

All these issues, and others of personal relevance, may be addressed within the problem-solving framework. Additional support from job clubs, where groups of people may meet to participate in skill training sessions, problem solve with one another, and gain day-to-day support for their efforts have provided high levels of successful job rehabilitation (Azrin & Basalel, 1980). Jacobs and colleagues (1983) have reported that two-thirds of people attending such a program were able to sustain employment for at least six months. In many services however, an assessment of an individual's ability to carry out the many tasks needed to obtain and hold down a job does not take place, nor is any training provided to help the person to acquire these skills. Lack of success in obtaining a job is then interpreted as poor motivation or as evidence of a severe disability which cannot be changed. We have found that if appropriate training is provided, most people can find some form of rewarding occupation in their own community.

Home-based rehabilitation addresses the needs for supportive work activities of the entire household. In some cases it may make more sense for a caregiving mother or wife to return to work, while the more disabled person they are supporting takes over home-making roles, as was the case in the example of the truck driver above. Return to work after a long period at home may be eased by applying the same skill training and problem solving for the carer. Common concerns about leaving a disabled person at home alone may be eased by careful planning. In addition, such problem solving may facilitate changes in traditional role behaviour of other members of the household, who may be willing to assist in caring and household management, particularly when they too can receive training in those skills where they have major deficits. For example, Tom agreed to help out with evening meals. His wife planned to train him to prepare a range of basic meals. This proved rather difficult for her as she set high standards of kitchen hygiene and had difficultly not taking over when Tom made a mess. However, after achieving basic skills, Tom became very interested in cooking and attended evening classes in Chinese and then Italian cookery!

The integrated community approach facilitates access to a wide range of neighbourhood work opportunities that are not considered in traditional programs. For example: Polly was a 32-year-old single woman, who lived alone and enjoyed caring for a menagerie of animals. She was given the task of brainstorming all possible work activities she might consider within her neighbourhood and developed the following list:

job centre	animal hospital
job club	assisting veterinarian
looking in newspapers	practising interviews
voluntary groups	neighbourhood patrol
church	shopping for elderly
gardening	lawn care
cleaning	walking dogs
pet care	night classes
assisting at schools	hospital visiting
baby sitting	cooking
cleaning litter	recycling cans/paper
running errands	making job enquiries
visiting businesses	work experience
conservation projects	guide dogs for the blind
surveys	delivering mail/leaflets
work for RSPCA	reading/getting ideas
becoming an artist	writing news for local paper
growing vegetables	decorating house

cutting hedges	growing seedlings
home typing	spinning lambswool
knitting	dressmaking

This illustrates the huge range of options available to people who are integrated into life in the community and the resources that exist there. Specialised sheltered work, like sheltered leisure (day care), tends to increase handicap, by limiting the scope of rehabilitation, as well as portraying people with mental disorders as a group who cannot benefit from participation in the resources the community provides. The special needs of people recovering from mental disorders are best served by being treated as ordinary citizens, who may need to reintegrate into the work-force in gradual steps, in a manner similar to that of a person who has suffered a heart disorder or any other major illness. Furthermore that person, in similar fashion, may never regain their former work capacity. Assisting people to gain access to the workplace is a crucial role for mental health therapists, as well as ensuring that they are not victims of discrimination.

Family care alternatives

While no alternative to living at home with family members has been demonstrated to provide a better environment in which to recover from mental disorders, there are occasions when, after extensive family-based training, a person experiencing persisting high levels of ambient stress may wish to seek a less stressful habitat within the community (Figure 8.2). Although there is no controlled research to support any family care alternatives, a range of supported housing options have been devised. These include:

Halfway houses or hostels: A residence that provides 24-hour professional support for a group of people recovering from mental disorders. Meals are usually provided, and residents are encouraged to participate in a range of counselling, work and daily living projects, under the daily supervision of the professional team. It is expected that residents will move on to independent living settings in the community.

Long-term group residences: These are residences for people with long-term severe disability who are provided with similar support and supervision to those living in long-stay hospital units. Expectations are low, and efforts at rehabilitation are minimal.

Co-operative apartments or group homes: These are houses or apartments shared by small groups of residents, who work together to create a family-like lifestyle. Training in living skills has usually been undertaken in a hospital or halfway house prior to this move. Regular visits are made from staff to provide support and supervision.

Foster care: Families are recruited in the community to provide foster care for people recovering from mental disorders, who cannot be managed effectively by their natural carers. This may be used for short-term respite or for long-term residence. Professional support and training is provided on a regular basis.

The aim of all these alternatives is to provide a home-like alternative for residents. The absence of research prevents any clear discussion on their relative merits. However, it is clear that it is the quality of the interpersonal environment that is provided that is crucial rather than the structure of the residence. Most families find it impossible to cope with more than one person who is vulnerable to a major health problem living in a the household at any given time. Therefore, it is necessary to have extraordinary stress management skills to enable a group of people with high vulnerability to mental disorders to live in a community setting without frequent major crises. Thus, it is probably advisable to support living settings where one vulnerable person is cared for by one or more less vulnerable people. Of all the alternatives cited above only the foster care arrangement meets that goal. One follow-up study of long-term fostering in Canada supported the feasibility of this method, but the results in terms of reduced impairment and disability were not encouraging (Linn, 1981).

Until further research supports the value of alternatives to family care we believe that services should focus their resources on ensuring that effective support is provided to family carers, including close friends and neighbours who provide a family-style living. Where such carers have been fully integrated into the mental health service and trained in stress management and other relevant strategies, they have not merely provided a supportive environment, but their efforts have contributed to substantial reductions in impairment and disability, as well as personal benefits to themselves (Falloon, 1985). This outstanding resource has reduced the need for alternatives to a level where existing housing resources in the community can be employed for respite care, and where the majority of people moving out of family care are ready to move to more independent living, provided this is done in a carefully planned manner. However, regardless of where, or with whom, a person resides they will benefit from a home-based approach to their clinical management, preferably one that involves the key carers in their social habitat, whether these are relatives, friends, room-mates or neighbours.

Specific psychological strategies

In addition to family-based stress management and living skills training, several psychological strategies have been demonstrated as effective in reducing persistent impairment and disability associated with mental disorders. Several of these strategies have been described in Chapters 5 and 6. These included strategies for managing anxiety and depression, eating and sleep disorders, negative thought patterns, anger and aggression, compliance, suicidal thoughts, and persisting delusions and hallucinations. Two problems that were not addressed were motivational deficits and persistent cognitive deficits. These are of particular relevance when working with people with long-standing or severe disorders.

Motivational deficits

People who appear to have reduced drive to engage in constructive activity are often considered to have reduced levels of motivation, or 'negative' symptoms. The origins of these deficits are usually complex, with the effects of drug therapy, persisting cognitive and mood disorder, and lack of incentives all playing a part. Balancing drug treatment to minimise drug-related impairment, while maximising reductions in psychopathology is an important first step in the management of such states.

Regardless of the origins of reduced drive, operant strategies may be helpful in providing added motivation. Such a program involves clarifying the specific objects and activities a person finds most rewarding and employing these to reinforce efforts to undertake specific small steps towards achieving realistic personal goals. Of course, setting goals with severely disabled people may be a lengthy process, particularly when the gap between their expected and current levels of performance is wide. However, morale is greatly enhanced when the disabled person can envisage a long-term way to bridge this gap in a series of manageable steps.

An example was Joanna, a 28 year-old woman, who was keen to return to her secretarial job after a schizophrenic episode. She heard persisting voices that interrupted her ability to concentrate for more than a minute or two. As a result she spent most of her time lying in bed or listening to music. All efforts to further reduce her symptoms through drug therapy proved unsuccessful. Her therapist and mother helped her to set a short-term goal of typing letters for her brothers' business. It was agreed that she would be paid for each completed letter. In addition, she could choose rewards of specified food treats, time listening to music or watching television, for each five- minute period of effort attempting to perform this task. Initially, even this brief period proved too difficult and it was reduced to two minutes. She found that she could concentrate for this period and that her excellent typing skills were retained and she made minimal errors. Gradually she began to be able to concentrate for longer periods. As this occurred her incentive program was adjusted so that she agreed to carry out more tasks before receiving her chosen rewards. Within three months she was able to take over most of the clerical work for her brother's small catering business. However, her need for frequent breaks made returning to work in an office setting still some way off.

Studies of the effectiveness of individualised programs of operant strategies have shown considerable benefits when compared with traditional and supportive methods (Paul & Lentz, 1977; Baker et al, 1977). However, the application of group-oriented programs that are not designed to meet individual needs have proven less successful and tend to have only limited long-term benefits (Hall & Baker, 1986).

Cognitive skills training

This strategy has been devised to assist people with persisting cognitive disabilities, such as concentration and attention disorders, recall and recognition problems, misinterpretation of social cues, and problem-solving deficits. Although at present these methods

remain in the research and development phase, the early reports
suggest that they may be an important advance in the management
of cognitive disability associated with schizophrenia and other
disorders (Brenner, 1988). In the absence of professionals trained to
apply these new cognitive training methods, therapists may use
training methods that take account of the cognitive deficits. For
example, where attention span is low, training may need to occur in
a series of brief segments (sometimes no more than 2–3 minutes
long) with breaks between, rather than continuous hour-long sessions. Where recall is limited, therapists may need to repeat themselves many times, check on what has been recalled, and use
straightforward written materials as back-up. As with all integrated
care, the approach is tailored to the specific strengths and weaknesses of each participant.

Continuing integrated case management

Integrated clinical management has the major goal of ensuring that
all people suffering disabling, or potentially disabling mental disorders receive optimal combinations of biomedical, psychological
and social interventions until they show evidence of sustained
recovery from all impairment, disability and handicap associated
with their disorders, including any morbidity associated with informal caregiving. Case management resides within a team that is
integrated into the primary care services of the community (see
Figure 8.6). Within this multidisciplinary team, comprising nurse
therapists, social workers, occupational therapists, psychologists,
community general and obstetric nurses, psychiatrists and family
practitioners, one professional is designated the key worker for each
case. This person is trained to administer in a competent manner the
full range of assessment methods, as well as carer-based stress
management, living skills training, and specific psychological strategies. With complex cases therapeutic interventions are usually
provided by several members of the team, with the key worker
coordinating these efforts, which at times may approach the intensity provided in crisis care, i.e. daily interventions extending over
several hours. It is crucial that sufficient staff are available for long-
term management at all times, and that this work is given a high
priority. In order to provide integrated clinical management to all

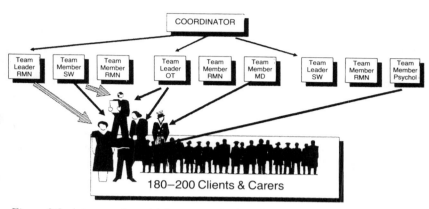

Figure 8.6. A teamwork model for community-based mental health care.

who need this, it may be necessary for staff to work some evenings and weekends on a flexible schedule. Regular review of progress on standardised ratings provides feedback to the team, and the focus on rewarding effort more than achievement provides support for the team and the key worker in particular. Intensive training is provided in weekly half-day workshops, as well as in detailed case supervision with participating therapists. Therapists use the skill training and stress management methods to practice their own interventions and to cope with their own stresses. In this manner long-term support is sustained and morale is maintained among the professional team.

A similar approach is used to sustain the continuing efforts of patients and their carers. While developing competence in living skills, achieving optimal drug therapy or acquiring understanding about the disorder may be the initial goals of intervention, there is no guarantee that such benefits will be maintained. Maintenance of function at any given level and the prevention of deterioration in role performance requires regular and often intensive intervention. Furthermore, having achieved an improved quality of life usually leads to setting further personal goals. It is important for people who work with the long-term disabled to be aware that progress may be slow, with periods of significant progress interspersed with quiescent periods when little benefit seem to accrue from continued therapeutic effort. The tendency to impose one's own goals to expedite progress is probably best avoided at these times when progress plateaus. It is equally important not to err on the side of

becoming complacent or discouraged and not provide the necessary clinical interventions to ensure that people achieve their maximum potential and that their quality of life is enhanced as far as
possible.

In practice this approach often means that skills already taught,
information already provided and strategies already tried have to be
revised again and again. Less frequently, prolonged lack of progress
may require a substantial change in direction, with introduction of
new strategies. More often impatient therapists dismiss potentially
effective strategies too readily on the grounds that they have not
shown dramatic benefits or as having been 'tried already' and have
not resulted in achievement of the desired goals. In these cases the
problem is frequently that interventions have not been paced cor-
rectly or sufficient account has not been taken of the effects of factors
such as cognitive impairment which may interfere with the person's
ability to process and retain information and skills. Careful analysis
of why particular interventions have not worked is essential to
ensure that interventions with proven effectiveness are used to
maximum effect.

In other cases an examination of why skills learned have not
been maintained will cast light on other relevant factors, such as
the lack of opportunity to practice skills, lack of reinforcement or
success experiences when using the skills, or lack of feedback from
others in the family or in the community. The approach taken at
this point will be linked to this reassessment and will aim to resolve
some of the difficulties encountered or may be directed more
towards family members or other significant people in the person's
social network.

An example was the case of Pete, who had become very skilled at how to
perform job interviews. His therapist had used repeated role-play practice
with modelling and coaching to prepare him for any situation that might arise.
However, these skills deteriorated because he had not yet had the
opportunity to use them, as he had not yet been called to an interview. An
assessment of the situation revealed that his job-seeking skills were poor and
he was too anxious to visit job centres. Skill training was adjusted to focus on
job finding. Pete learnt the various ways in which jobs are advertised, and
then was accompanied to the job centre after he had rehearsed how to ask
for the information he required. When he finally was given an interview he
decided to treat this as another practice session. Before the interview he
brushed up his skills with further role-played practice. He was very pleased
with his performance in the interview, which was much easier than he had

expected. Although he did not get the job he was delighted that he was placed on a reserve list ahead of several more experienced applicants.

In other cases, attention may focus on integrating carers in the plan. For example:

Wendy had ongoing difficulties with personal hygiene which caused great concern to her family and of which they were very critical. Following a careful program of setting realistic achievable goals, this improved and there were no longer any problems in this area. However, while members of her family were involved in the program initially, when Wendy's hygiene improved they did not continue to remind her of what she needed to do, nor did they compliment her when she had actually showered and had taken care of her personal appearance. After a few weeks, there had been a deterioration and Wendy was again refusing to wash.

Intervention at this stage focussed on involving the family to a greater extent in the program, and of looking with them at ways in which they could continue to take interest and compliment Wendy on the efforts she had made, especially when they no longer perceived her personal hygiene to be a problem.

Conclusion

It is concluded that integrated long-term management combines optimal drug therapy with extensive skills training and specific psychosocial strategies. All this is based within the context of comprehensive social casework to ensure that housing, finances, work and recreational resources in the community are accessed fully, without discrimination. Further, the carer-based management system facilitates stress management, and integrates informal carers into all aspects of the program in a manner that ensures that their personal needs are met and the quality of their lives enhanced as well as those of the disabled for whom they care. Continuous monitoring of progress towards personal goals of all participants, their stress and coping, as well as fluctuations in impairments, disabilities and handicaps guide the therapy team to adapt intervention strategies to the changing needs of each individual. Education and training are crucial components of this approach at all levels – patients, carers, community resources, primary care and mental health specialists. Above all, intensive intervention ceases only when sustained full recovery of functioning has been achieved.

Thanks to Bridget Lake, Occupational Therapist for help with the case examples used in this chapter.

References

Azrin N.H. & Basalel V. (1980) *Job club counselor's manual: a behavioral approach to vocational counseling.* University Park Press, Baltimore.

Baker R.D. & Hall J.N. (1983) *REHAB: a multipurpose assessment instrument for long-stay patients.* Vine Publishing, Aberdeen.

Baker R.D., Hall J.N., Hutchinson K. & Bridge G. (1977) Symptom changes in chronic schizophrenic patients on a token economy: a controlled experiment. *British Journal of Psychiatry,* **131**, 381.

Bellack A.S., Hersen, M. & Himmelhoch J.M. (1983) A comparison of social skills training, pharmacotherapy and psychotherapy for depression. *Behaviour, Research & Therapy,* **21**, 101–107.

Brenner H.D. (1988) On the importance of cognitive disorders in treatment and rehabilitation. In J.S. Strauss, W. Boker & H.D. Brenner (Eds.) *Psychosocial treatment of schizophrenia.* Huber-Verlag, New York.

Carpenter W.T., Heinrichs D.W. & Hanlon T.E. (1987) A comparative trial of pharmacologic strategies in schizophrenia. *American Journal of Psychiatry,* **144**, 1466–1470.

Falloon I.R.H. (1985) *Family management of schizophrenia.* Johns Hopkins University Press, Baltimore.

Falloon I.R.H., Watt D.C. & Shepherd M. (1978) The social outcome of patients in a trial of long-term continuation therapy in schizophrenia: pimozide vs. fluphenazine. *Psychological Medicine,* **8**, 265–274.

Goldstrom I. & Manderscheid R. (1982) The chronically mentally ill: a descriptive analysis from the uniform client data instrument. *Journal of Community Support Services,* **2**, 4.

Hall J.N. & Baker R.D. (1986) Token economies and schizophrenia; a review. In A. Kerr & R.P. Snaith (Eds.) *Contemporary issues in schizophrenia.* Gaskell Press, London.

Hogarty G.E., Goldberg S.C., Schooler N.R. & Ulrich R.F. (1974) The collaborative study group: Drug and sociotherapy in the aftercare of schizophrenic patients. II. Two-year relapse rates. *Archives of General Psychiatry,* **31**, 603–608.

Hogarty G.E., Schooler N.R., Ulrich R.F., Mussare F. & Herron E. (1979) Fluphenazine and social therapy in the aftercare of schizophrenic patients: relapse analysis of a two-year controlled trial. *Archives of General Psychiatry,* **36**, 1283–1294.

Jacobs H., Donahoe P. & Falloon I.R.H. (1983) Rehabilitation of the chronic schizophrenic. In T. Backer, L. Pan & C.L. Vash (Eds.) *Annual review of rehabilitation, 1983.* Springer-Verlag, New York.

Kane J.M., Woerner M. & Sarentakos S. (1986) Depot neuroleptics: a comparative review of standard intermediate and low-dose regimens. *Journal of Clinical Psychiatry*, **47**(5), (Suppl), 30–33.

Lamb H.R. (1979) New asylums in the community. *Archives of General Psychiatry*, **36**, 129–134.

Liberman R.P., DeRisi W.J. & Mueser K.T. (1989) *Social skills training for psychiatric patients*. Pergamon, New York.

Linn M.W. (1981) Can foster care survive? *New Directions in Mental Health Services*, **11**, 35.

Marder S.R., Van Putten T., Mintz J. et al. (1988) Low- and conventional-dose maintenance therapy with fluphenazine decanoate. *Archives of General Psychiatry*, **44**, 518–521.

Paul G.C. & Lentz R.J. (1977) *Psychosocial treatment of chronic mental patients*. Harvard University Press, Cambridge MA.

Schooler N.R., Levine J. Severe J.B., Brauzer B. & DiMascio A. (1980) Prevention of relapse in schizophrenia: an evaluation of fluphenazine decanoate. *Archives of General Psychiatry*, **37**, 16–24.

Wallace C.J. (1990) *Independent living skills survey (ILSS)*. Clinical Research Center for Schizophrenia & Psychiatric Rehabilitation, Los Angeles.

Wallace C.J. & Liberman R.P. (1985) Social skills training for patients with schizophrenia: a controlled clinical trial. *Psychiatry Research*, **15**, 239–247.

Wing J.K., Bennett D.H. & Denham J. (1964) The industrial rehabilitation of long-stay schizophrenia patients. *Medical Research Council Memo No.42*. H.M.S.O: London.

9
Assessment of benefits and costs of the service to the community

The last component in the development of an integrated mental health service is the evaluation of outcome of the service in meeting the needs of the community. This evaluation must address the following issues:

1 *Accessibility*. To demonstrate that the optimal service is being provided to all the people in the defined community who are experiencing mental disorders in a time and manner that maximises effectiveness.
2 *Acceptability*. To demonstrate that the consumers find the service delivery acceptable, with the benefits to them balancing or outweighing the personal costs.
3 *Accountability*. To demonstrate that the service is effective and efficient in reducing impairment, disability and handicap associated with all the expressed needs for mental health services to the community.
4 *Adaptability*. To demonstrate that the service is able to adapt to the changing patterns of needs of the community, including the differing needs of people during different phases of their disorders.

In this chapter we will describe a system of assessing these four requirements that has been developed and employed to achieve these aims within the framework of everyday clinical practice.

Accessibility

Any service that is successful in meeting the needs of a community must ensure that the state-of-the-art clinical management is received by all people who have need for that service. The ability of a service to reach all cases of people with mental disorders in the community, particularly those who will benefit most from modern clinical management, is an important measure of its success. However, as we have discussed earlier, much mental disorder, even in its most severe manifestations, remains hidden. This appears largely due to the ineffectiveness of screening at a primary care level, as well as to the reluctance of people experiencing mental disorders and their carers to seek consultation for those mental disorders. Thus, it may be assumed that successful efforts to enhance accessibility to mental health care might be reflected in a rising number of cases being referred to the specialist service. However, many family practitioners have considerable skills in the clinical management of mental disorders, and others may acquire greater skill and confidence as a result of the tutoring they receive from the practice-based team. For this reason the only valid index of accessibility would be derived from a community survey that examined the proportion of people in the community experiencing mental disorders who were receiving optimal clinical management for their disorders, from all existing services. As accessibility improved, this proportion would be expected to increase, until the point where all cases were diagnosed appropriately and receiving adequate clinical management and where the clinical population closely approximated that uncovered by community surveys (Strathdee et al, 1990). Unfortunately, the resources needed to conduct such surveys are considerable, so that it is likely that estimates will have to be made from examination of the cases detected and receiving treatment in each family practice. A further problem is the proportion of people who do not have mental disorders, yet are in receipt of mental health management, at times to their detriment. The proportion of such cases often mistakenly diagnosed as having mental disorders should be minimal in an efficient mental health service. However, in the absence of alternative psychosocial counselling services, a mental health service may feel able to volunteer a small proportion of its resources to provide a community service to those distressed and demoralised people, who may be suffering similar disabilities and handicaps to those with actual mental disorders. However, at no time should management of such cases prevent any person suffering from a mental disorder obtaining optimal clinical management.

Extensive surveys of people attending family practices have been conducted using questionnaires, such as the General Health Questionnaire (Goldberg & Blackwell, 1970). Such surveys have been

Table 9.1. *Characteristics of population assessed by an integrated mental health service during a 12-month period*

Number referred	376	(100%)
Sex		
Female	261	(69%)
Male	115	(31%)
Age	36	(range 14–69)
Marital status		
Married	235	(63%)
Widowed	13	(3%)
Divorced	34	(9%)
Single	84	(22%)
Education		
University	37	(10%)
High school completed	237	(63%)
High school attendance	59	(16%)
No high school	32	(9%)
Currently employed (including students, homemakers)	301	(80%)
Health status		
Current physical disorder	85	(23%)
Previous mental disorder	138	(37%)
Family history of mental disorder	100	(27%)

useful in detecting minor mental disorders, but of limited value in uncovering the hidden morbidity due to schizophrenia and other disabling but less common major disorders. Despite the limitations of such questionnaire surveys they have the advantage of being very straightforward and easy to administer (Newman et al, 1990). Thus, an annual questionnaire survey conducted at each family practice in the community that established the proportion of 'cases' identified in this manner, who were receiving the appropriate levels of mental health care, would provide a useful guide to accessibility of the integrated service.

We have not yet established such an approach. A much cruder index has been employed that has examined the requests for specialist consultations with 'new' cases that have been made since the advent of the integrated service. These have risen from around 150 per 100,000 population to around 1200 per 100,000 annually (see Tables 9.1 & 9.2). However, the proportion of specialist assessments on people who did not have mental disorders has increased from around 10% to almost 50%. Most of this increase is made up of

Table 9.2. *DSM-III-R diagnosis of people assessed by an integrated mental health service during 12 months*

Diagnosis	First assessment	Reassessment/ moved to area	Total	No. per 100,000
Anxiety disorders	54	17	71	213
Adjustment disorders	38	25	63	189
Somatisation, etc.	19	6	25	75
Dysthymic disorders	6	6	10	30
Eating disorders	6	4	10	30
Major affective disorders	4	3	7	21
Schizophrenic disorders	0	5[a]	5	3
Organic disorders	3	1	4	12
Other mental disorders	0	2	2	6
Psychosocial disorders				
1° substance abuse	11	3	14	42
2° substance abuse	11	5	16	48
1° personality disorders	7	0	7	21
2° personality disorders	10	11	21	63
Sexual dysfunction	5	2	7	21
Family/marital/work	76	27	103	309
No disorder	36	11	47	

Note: [a] Four cases were referred from neighbouring services in order to receive specialist clinical management.

requests from five of the 18 family practitioners, who have opted to have the mental health team screen cases rather than attempt to do this themselves. Indeed, less than one in four of the requests for specialist attention from one family practitioner were found to have mental disorders. On the other hand 90% of the requests of another family practitioner had mental disorders. Such data is all too readily interpreted as indicating a lack of screening ability in the former, and exceptional ability in the latter. However, this is not necessarily so. In close-knit communities family practitioners gain reputations for their expertise in different areas. The doctor who requested help with mainly non-psychiatric cases 'specialised' in assisting people in marital and social difficulties. Thus, most of his requests were for management of psychosocial distress and family breakdown. The second doctor, had completed considerable psychiatric training and attracted people with mental disorders, for whom she sought early assistance from the multidisciplinary specialists.

It may be concluded, tentatively, that the integrated community service made it easier for people to gain access to specialist mental health assessments and integrated treatment. This increase was most marked for those people who presented to their family practitioners in distressed emotional states, but there was an associated three- to four-fold increase in the detection of mental disorders. Nevertheless, this rate left around 90% of cases of mental disorder probably unrecognised (when compared with Goldberg & Huxley, 1980; see also Figure 1.2). But this figure is undoubtedly reduced by the manner in which the integrated service always attempted to assess not merely the presenting patient, but also all key family members or other carers. This additional screening contributed to a substantial increase in detection of both minor and major disorders, and often led to friends and neighbours coming forward to seek help for themselves or people that they in turn cared for. Over a period of 5 years it was estimated that the service had screened at least 1 in 5 adults living in the community. This led to a doubling of the number of people with long-term disability associated with major mental disorders who were provided with access to intensive rehabilitation programs. Several previously undetected severe cases of schizophrenia and obsessive-compulsive disorder were assessed and treated for the first time. Previous efforts by their family practitioners to seek assistance in their care had failed when these people had been unable or unwilling to seek hospital-based care, compulsory treatment was not indicated, and home-based alternatives not available.

However, despite these notable successes, it was still evident that most mental disorders remained hidden when our figures were compared to those found in community surveys (Dilling & Weyerer, 1984; Myers et al, 1984). This led to the initiation of two further projects that aimed to increase detection of mental disorders, particularly those associated with high levels of disability. The first, was the strategy to enhance early detection of schizophrenic and associated disorders that has been described earlier (Chapter 4, p. 111). The second, involved a review of all people prescribed minor tranquillising drugs, either for short-term or long-term use. We found remarkably few cases in either category. Most family practitioners told us that they now preferred to send people to the mental health therapists rather than prescribe tranquillisers or sedatives. The difference between writing a prescription and completing our request for consultation form was minimal in terms of time and effort, and this combined with immediate response to requests for consultation, undoubtedly contributed to this change in practice. Special training enabled all therapists to carry out drug withdrawal programs for people wishing to stop long-term prescription drug use. One of our family practitioner colleagues provided considerable assistance to this training, by devising an ingenious method of gradual withdrawal from benzodiazepines (Clark, 1989). This involved transferring people to diazepam suspension, that they diluted after each dose by adding an amount of water equal to the amount of the suspension they had taken for that dose. This method has proven extremely effective in minimising withdrawal reactions, and illustrates the mutual assistance provided by this integrated approach.

Further concerns about accessibility were associated with the predominance of women assessed, diagnosed and subsequently treated, and the lack of major affective disorders, particularly depression. Although community surveys do detect a slight excess of female cases, we had expected that the ratio of cases detected with the integrated approach would be more equally distributed between the sexes than the 2:1 we observed. This ratio decreased to 3:2 when mild cases (Clinical Global Impression Scale (CGI) < 3; see p. 272) were excluded. Efforts have been underway to examine ways to enhance screening of men in the population. These include, having mental health therapists available throughout the evening family practice clinics, and conducting assessments at weekends.

The extremely low incidence of major depressive episodes is possibly a consequence of the early detection and intervention provided by the integrated service. A large proportion of potential cases were treated successfully at an early stage in their depressive episodes, and were classified as adjustment disorders. A similar phenomenon has been noted with the functional psychoses, with very few cases meeting the stringent criteria for schizophrenic disorders. These observations must be subject to controlled evaluation before they can be viewed as anything more than artefacts of the classification system, and undoubtedly cases of severe disorders remain undetected, despite our efforts.

Audit and quality assurance

It is usually assumed that any case that obtains access to a service immediately receives optimal management for their problems. However, that assumption is seldom tested, even in centres of excellence. We adopted a series of strategies to ensure that every person who accessed the specialist part of the service received optimal clinical management.

Standardised assessment

Every therapist, regardless of professional discipline, completed an identical assessment for every case, that was coded systematically and placed on a computer file for record keeping. This included information on each person's vulnerability, medical and social history, as well as diagnosis, levels of impairment, disability and handicap, carer stress, treatment goals and problems, management plan and progress indices. Additional detailed note keeping was minimal and for therapists' personal reference only. Therapists received training in completing these semi-structured assessments, which formed the basis for subsequent supervision and quality assurance.

Initial team review

Every new consultation was reviewed by the multidisciplinary team at the weekly family practice meeting. Key issues from the assessment were highlighted, and the therapist's provisional management plan discussed, and approved by the entire team. Prior approval had been sought from the patients and carers. Where uncertainties remained, second opinions from other members of the professional team were sought, or from other specialised agencies. This often involved conjoint assessments of aspects of biomedical, psychological or social factors. It should be recalled that every case received integrated clinical management that encompassed each of these components in varying degrees. For problems where specific strategies have been validated as having specific benefits, the optimal strategy or combination of strategies was chosen for the initial intervention. In those disorders where no specific approaches had yet been validated, the team assisted the therapist in devising an experimental approach that applied existing knowledge to the development of a management plan. This plan included outcome measures in order to facilitate a rigorous review of its effectiveness. Regardless of the management plan, every case was considered an

Table 9.3. *Review of progress*

Target problem rating (Falloon, 1985)
Level of impairment from mental disorder: Clinical Global Impression (Guy, 1976)
Level of psychosocial disability: Charing Cross Health Index (Rosser & Kind, 1978)
Level of carer stress: Global Family Burden Scale (Falloon, 1985)

experimental case study, and validated strategies were tailored to the unique assets and deficits of each case.

Case supervision

The leader of each family practice team assumed responsibility for ensuring that optimal clinical management was provided for each case at each phase of their condition. This entailed providing specific guidance for each therapist in the team, and ensuring that nobody attempted to perform any aspect of management that they were not competent to undertake. Where a specific assessment or treatment strategy was beyond the competence of the key worker, they were responsible for seeking the assistance of another member of the service who had the necessary competence. Wherever possible that expert conducted the procedure in conjoint sessions with the key worker, who may be trained subsequently to conduct some or all of the procedure themselves. Occasionally specialist help may be needed from experts outside the service. Once again every attempt was made to conduct this work in a conjoint way to facilitate training. Every member of the service was expected to obtain regular case supervision from other members of the team, no matter how experienced or senior.

Subsequent team review

As well as defining the methods of case supervision, the initial review also defined the date for subsequent review of the progress of the clinical management. Review of progress focussed on evidence of reduction in impairment, disability and handicap as indicated by changes in the standardised ratings, as well as those of targeted problems and goals (see Table 9.3). A lack of expected progress was analysed in terms of the effectiveness of assessment and treat-ment strategies. The efforts of the therapist are clearly acknowl-edged, despite limited achievement, and the team used the problem-solving approach to develop further plans to overcome the difficulties. Thus, it was the *methods* that were subjected to criticism, not the therapists.

The frequency of review was tailored to each case, with some cases receiving intensive care being reviewed daily. The management of long-term cases in the rehabilitation phase were subjected to com-prehensive review every three months. This review was similar to that provided for cases in the early phase of intervention, but in addition included standardised ratings of community tenure, work activity, environmental stress, and details of all services received. Clinical review considered all aspects of current needs, including a comprehensive review of any drug strategies and the emergence of side effects. Constant rehabilitation efforts continued at least until all evidence of impairment, disability and handicap associated with mental disorder had been absent continuously for at least 24 months. Even when people decided that they did not wish to participate in any further active rehabilitation, the therapist negotiated a plan with them that they continue to participate in this monitoring process. This ensured that contact was maintained and the tran-sition back to active intervention was facilitated at any time when deterioration may begin, or the person's renewed interest in further reducing any residual morbidity may lead them to re-enter the active rehabilitation program. It was recognised that breaks in active intervention could be used in a constructive manner, and that this did not need to lead to withdrawal from the service. On occasions these plans involved periods of monitoring primarily by family practitioners and carers.

These strategies have been remarkably successful at ensuring that every case that received specialised management from the service was provided with optimal interventions throughout the various phases of their disorder. Unfortunately we have been unable to carry out similar audit of the quality of clinical management that has been implemented by our primary care colleagues. Without such a review it is difficult to make any claims for the quality of mental health care provided to the whole community.

Acceptability

An effective service must be able to demonstrate that it provides clinical management in a manner that is acceptable to all consumers. Unless the benefits they acquire from the service outweigh the costs, both emotional and/or economic, it is unlikely that consumers will continue to access the service, and a high drop-out rate will result. In addition to the rate of drop outs, indices of acceptability may include the rate of uptake of management and levels of satisfaction expressed by patients and carers. The satisfaction expressed with the service by staff and other professional agencies in the community may prove valuable.

Uptake of interventions offered

This refers to the proportion of cases who are successfully engaged in clinical management. There is evidence that delays in obtaining initial appointments for specialised mental health assessment tend to reduce uptake (Kluger & Karras, 1983). Further evidence suggests that the level of agreement between consumers and professionals in defining the initial goals of intervention programs determines the uptake (Falloon & Talbot, 1982). A service that attempts to provide assessment and treatment in the location and time chosen primarily by the consumer, and with minimal delays, may be expected to prove more acceptable than one where formal appointments are made without consultation with the consumers, in anxiety-provoking clinical settings, and often with waits of several weeks. Thus, it might be expected that the integrated mental health service approach might show an improved rate of uptake of specialist consultations. The uptake rate in the Buckingham Project was around 95%. This compares with rates of between 50 and 75% in hospital-based mental health outpatient services (Chen, 1991). Wherever possible, non-attenders were interviewed in order to determine their reasons for avoiding specialist consultation. The main reason given was that their family practitioner had recommended the consultation without explaining what this entailed and the potential benefits. In all cases a mental health therapist was not available in the practice at the time of primary care screening. In no case was a clear need for specialist mental health management evident at the time they were contacted, and several people commented that they had obtained the help they sought from their contact with the family practitioner.

Two-thirds of all initial assessments were completed within one week of the request for consultation, and over 90% completed within three weeks. A small proportion of people who were suspected of having mental disorders were reluctant to complete assessments. An assertive approach was employed to ensure that they were engaged. This often involved problem solving with their carers and family practitioners over several weeks until the reluctant person agreed to meet with a mental health therapist. This persistent non-coercive approach enabled all such cases to eventually complete mental health screening, on occasions up to three months after the initial request had been made.

Withdrawal from clinical management

A further measure of the acceptability of a service is the rate at which people who are initially engaged in clinical management subsequently withdraw from major components of the clinical management contract. This covers a range from suboptimal compliance with treatment strategies to refusal of all contact with the service. Measures of adherence to treatment regimens, particularly those that involve combinations of strategies, are very difficult to devise, but are crucial estimates of the quality of the service, and of the competence of individual therapists. Many services pay relatively little attention to this important aspect and regard non-compliers and drop outs as a reflection of the lack of motivation of the clients rather than ineffectiveness of the service.

The integrated service attempts to develop team-work between the patients, carers and therapists, whereby each aspect of the clinical management plan is contracted in a mutually agreed manner, with constant review of the benefits and costs to the consumers. In addition, compliance training was an major component of all long-term management. This was based upon the expectation that the perceived benefits of most prophylactic interventions would appear less that the personal costs for many people from time to time. It might be assumed that this client-centred approach might lead to a high level of adherence to optimal management. This was certainly true of cases receiving long-term management for major

Table 9.4. *Incomplete treatment one year after initial consultation*

Requests for assessments	376	(100%)
Refused assessment	12	(3%)
Refused treatment	24	(7%)
Discontinued treatment prematurely	81	(22%)
(A) psychosocial problems only	59	(16%)
(B) mental disorders	22	(6%)
Referred to more appropriate agencies	21	(6%)
Needed treatment after 3 months	112	(30%)
Continued treatment after 12 months	10	(3%)

disorders, where optimal adherence to drug and psychosocial management was very high. Over a two-year period no cases dropped out of management. Two cases (out of 72) did not adhere to optimal regimens. One male patient was reluctant to take continued neuroleptic drugs after his marriage broke up. He attributed the break up to sexual dysfunction associated with the drug therapy, despite the fact that this problem had been resolved several months before his wife left him and moved in with a neighbour. Intermittent medication was contracted, but proved ineffective. Extensive therapy was provided to develop a mutually acceptable drug regimen, with limited success, before the patient accepted an offer of more appropriate housing outside the area. A second long-term case was reluctant to adhere to the combined drug and psychological management recommended for her dysthymic state. She was fiercely independent and constantly studied books describing alternative therapies for depressive disorders and was able to debate the merits of various unvalidated approaches in a forceful manner. After more than two years of suboptimal therapy she finally participated in a course of cognitive-behavioural therapy combined with a monoamine oxidase inhibitor drug that led to rapid and complete recovery from her impairments.

Evidence to support the acceptability of the targeted clinical management offered to new cases is less impressive (Table 9.4). Those cases who withdrew from therapy prematurely without the mutual consent of the therapists, often appeared to have reached a point where they reported having obtained sufficient benefits to be able to manage without formal therapy sessions. Because all of our therapeutic approaches encouraged self-efficacy, such decisions to withdraw prematurely were not infrequently regarded as evidence for the success of the regimen. Where team review considered that the inadequate intervention had been provided and there was a high risk that the patient's disorder would deteriorate or recur unless further specialised treatment was provided, assertive efforts were made to re-engage patients and carers.

The consumers' view

Assessment of the consumers' perceptions of the service they receive may provide feedback to assist in improving its acceptability. However, the manner in which such surveys are conducted will have a major effect on the results. Clearly effective medicine does not have to taste good to prove highly efficacious, and not all medicine that tastes good is effective. Thus, it is crucial not to devise a mental health service entirely around the concept of pleasing the consumer. However, certain standards of professional behaviour should always be adhered to, such as punctuality, respect for clients, explanations for intervention procedures, rapport, or availability at times of crisis.

We conducted several independent surveys of consumers of the integrated service. The most detailed was a comparative interview study of people receiving treatment for depressive episodes in three services in the Oxford region (Taylor, 1989). The integrated approach obtained higher ratings from consumers than the two hospital-based community services on each of the following items:

help with benefits
talking and getting help from neighbours about problems i.e. less stigmatised
preferred outpatient appointments at family practice
mental health professionals involving them in treatment decisions
support from mental health team
given information about depression
family members understanding of depression
getting crisis help quickly
getting professional help for their depression
able to continue working
lower need for mental hospital care

Overall the ratings of the integrated service consumers were higher than the other services, significantly so when compared with the Oxford City service. Whereas most of the therapy was provided by nurse therapists in the integrated approach, the solitary consultant psychiatrist was the main therapist in the other two services.

A second questionnaire survey of 32 people who had completed early intervention was conducted by one of our nurse therapists, whilst she was seconded to a training course (Birch, 1990). Only one person made a rating of 'poor' or 'very poor' on any of the seven five-point scales (ranging from very good to very poor) that surveyed the response to various aspects of the clinical management. Thus, 99% of ratings indicated satisfaction with the service received, 81% either 'good' or 'very good'. A further series of questions on the professional standards demonstrated similarly high standards of acceptability. A surprising finding was that the highest satisfaction scores were reported where a male therapist was treating a female, and the lowest where a female therapist was treating a female. This contrasted with the view held by many family practitioners that the service needed more female therapists to treat female consumers.

Several positive comments were made about the therapists and the strategies they employed. One person commented that 'it was always referred to as my treatment and I could decide where I wanted it to go'. Another remarked 'I didn't know about this service until desperation gave me the courage to speak with my doctor. He is a very caring and astute doctor. Other people are perhaps not so lucky. I wonder how these people get help? How accessible are you? Thank you for being there for me and I hope the service will long continue to help and support others'.

A third study examined the satisfaction of people and their carers in the long-term program. Forty-four sufferers of long-term anxiety, major affective and schizophrenic disorders were interviewed, as well as their carers. Of these 91% were satisfied with the service overall; 98% of carers felt they had no difficulty in gaining the assistance of the team either at times of crisis, or at any other time they felt the need for guidance. However, 23% felt they had not received adequate guidance to fully manage their disorders without considerable continuing dependence on therapists. This was most evident with cases of anxiety disorders, where education tended to be less formal than that provided to sufferers and carers of the functional psychoses.

Comments on the most liked features of the integrated approach covered three recurrent themes: the accessibility of caring, competent therapists; the involvement of carers; and the team approach. Several people who had experienced changes in service delivery over many years commented on how much they wished the integrated approach had been available earlier. 'It's the best service I could imagine' remarked one carer; 'We get things we never expected. Regular checkups and really thorough, without any hassle', commented a patient. 'He's a great friend, who I feel I can say anything to and approach him at any time. We love to see him coming up the drive, even when I'm not at my best' was a typical comment about the consumers relationship with the therapists. 'The people listen to me. I told them I didn't think this heavy drug lark was much good, and they changed her to tablets. They keep her nice and steady' commented a husband who had cared for his wife for 30 years, with minimal support, since he had taken her home from a long-stay ward. 'He'd be in one of those hospitals now if it wasn't for the team. Even though he's still not well, we've all seen the slow improvement. I like the way they all work together with us even when there isn't much progress. In another year, maybe two, I'm sure he'll be more or less his old self again' was a comment from a mother on the long-term teamwork.

A few carers complained that they were not sufficiently involved in the management. In all these cases the patient had expressed clear wishes not to engage them despite constant requests from the therapists, and education about the expected benefits. Among the suggestions for improvement were the provision of childminding services; the revival of a relatives' and patients' support group that had been abandoned on account of a lack of participants (two carers and two patients only); more rapid response from family practitioners to requests for help; a telephone installed for emergencies (one family – although several had no phone, and relied on neighbours for emergency calls); improved timekeeping (two therapists).

It may be concluded that the integrated service was highly acceptable to consumers, who could identify few major needs that had not been met.

The professional view

Regular surveys of the family practitioners revealed a similarly high acceptance of the integrated service. The main aspects of the service that they preferred was the rapid response to consultation requests, accessibility, quality and professionalism of staff. Aspects that they would like to improve included the ability to request specific team members to assess cases, particularly the psychiatrists and women therapists. The facility already exists for the family practitioners to recommend specific assessors within the team framework. However, a few have continuing problems accepting the concept of a team approach, where every case is assessed and treated along biomedical and psychosocial lines. A few family practitioners were concerned about the adequacy of overnight management, suggesting that a higher level of staffing would be desirable on the odd occasions. Sixty per cent considered that the service was 'ideal', and the remainder thought that it would be if the overnight care was more intensive so that virtually no cases would need to be admitted to the inpatient psychiatric unit. Almost every family practitioner was eager to receive more formal training from the mental health professionals. Unfortunately, most found it difficult to attend formal seminars and workshops when these were arranged.

The mental health staff were generally pleased with the integrated approach (Caroline Hunt, personal communication). Without exception, they considered that they were working in a service that offered high quality clinical care to all members of the community. They considered the speed of response, accessibility, work with carers, and home-based intensive care especially beneficial. Several members expressed considerable enthusiasm for the use of quality assurance measures in clinical practice. A major asset from a professional standpoint was the regular and extensive training in proven techniques, the respect and autonomy given to each professional's competence, and the support experienced from the close multidisciplinary teamwork. A rating of personal satisfaction revealed that all members of the service were satisfied with their work, with 92% highly satisfied. Some concerns were expressed by less experienced staff about managing violence and suicide risks. These concerns were largely alleviated by providing further training in these areas. Throughout a five-year period only one violent incident involving a minor assault on a staff member occurred, and the rate of suicides over the same period was substantially lower than the national reported rates. Close teamwork among all disciplines as well as with patients, carers, family practitioners, and agencies, such as the local police and church groups enabled therapists to work with considerable confidence, even when faced with demanding circumstances. Above all, no staff member was ever expected to carry out any task that they were not trained to perform to a competent level. Furthermore, requests for assistance from any member of the team were met wherever possible. Where such requests appeared to be made by a person who was competent at performing the task, their anxiety or lack of confidence was examined in subsequent supervision, and they were assisted to overcome these problems, until they felt able to carry out the task in a more independent manner.

Burnout was not observed in the personnel associated with this service. However, colleagues in the primary care teams appeared to suffer a high degree of stress-related morbidity, and considerable assistance was provided for these colleagues. At times this involved consultation on the management of their services, as well as supportive interventions with their families.

Accountability

The most important measure of the value of a mental health service to a community is the efficiency with which it reduces the morbidity associated with all mental disorders. This includes not merely eliminating impairment, but also restoring patients and carers to full productive citizenship in the community. Thus, measures need to include impairment, disability and handicap.

Measures of efficiency also need to account for the cost of the service to the community. People living in a community will assess any new service in terms of both the added benefits it provides for citizens and the economic and personal cost of those benefits. In non-technological services such as mental health these costs reflect the use of professional therapeutic resources, and the effectiveness of the intervention strategies that are employed. Two methods of assessment have been devised. These are *cost-benefit analysis* and *cost-*

Table 9.5. Characteristics of cost–benefit and cost–effectiveness analyses

Cost–benefit analysis	Cost–effectiveness analysis
All costs and benefits are given monetary values (£)	Costs are given monetary values (£); benefits are valued in other units (e.g. clinical improvement; quality of life gained)
Allows comparison of different programmes (i.e. a health and a social service)	Allows comparison of programs with the same objectives only
Results are expressed in £ cost per £ benefit	Results are expressed in £ cost per unit gained (e.g. £ per life saved)
The inherent worth of a program can be measured (e.g. does £1m allocated to a health project produce more benefits than £1m given to a social project?)	Does not evaluate the inherent worth of a program (e.g. is £10,000 per year of improved quality of life worth while?)

effectiveness analysis. These methods, which are frequently misunderstood, will be reviewed briefly.

A *cost–benefit analysis* is conducted along monetary lines, with all costs and benefits being given monetary values, so that the results can be expressed in pounds of cost per pounds of benefit. In mental health care many of the benefits are not readily converted to monetary values and concern the quality of life of patients and carers. In such instances *cost-effectiveness analysis* is used to compare the monetary costs with units of benefits. Table 9.5 compares and contrasts these two approaches (see Cardin et al, 1985).

The effectiveness of a service may be gauged by the reductions in impairment, disability and handicap associated with mental disorder in the community it serves. Numerous measures have been validated to assess outcome in major research projects. However, many of these procedures are cumbersome, requiring extensive training for raters and complex methods of data analysis, that detract from their application in everyday clinical practice. We conducted a search for a set of rating scales that could be readily and reliably applied by clinicians from all disciplines within the constraints of busy clinical practice. In addition, the measures needed to be:

Table 9.6. *Clinical, Global Impressions Scale*

1 Normal, no mental illness at all
2 Borderline mentally ill
3 Mildly ill
4 Moderately ill
5 Markedly ill
6 Severely ill
7 Among the most extremely ill patients

Source: From Guy (1976).

1 Sensitive to change in morbidity levels.
2 Applicable to all mental disorders.
3 Repeatable at monthly intervals.
4 Acceptable to patients and carers in all phases of their disorders.
5 Able to provide specific, helpful feedback on treatment progress to clinicians.

Impairment

The level of impairment of each person's mental disorder was assessed on the *Clinical Global Impression Scale (CGI)* (Guy, 1976). This is a seven-point scale that assesses the overall severity of mental illness (see Table 9.6). It has been used extensively in drug trials and enables ratings to be made on a day-to-day basis. Comparisons can be made between people suffering different disorders. All staff were trained to make these ratings. Some difficulty was encountered initially in discriminating between distress and psychiatric impairment, and in deciding the borders between normal and abnormal anxiety or depressive phenomena. Because staff had all received training in the definition of symptoms using the clear guidelines provided for the Present State Examination (PSE) they were able to agree to employ similar criteria for their impairment ratings (in essence, impairment associated with a mental state was considered to be present when a person's reaction was out of proportion to the stress of their life circumstances, or would be expected to remain even when the adverse life circumstances that may have provoked the response had been resolved). Therapist ratings were reviewed at each team meeting and modified when a

Table 9.7. *Charing Cross Disability Scale*

8 Unconscious
7 Not in 8 but confined to bed
6 Not in 7 but confined to wheelchair or chair or able to move around in the home only with support from an assistant
5 Not in 6 but unable to undertake any paid employment. Unable to continue any education. Old people confined to home except for escorted outings and short walks and unable to do shopping. Housewives only able to perform a few simple tasks
4 Not in 5 but choice of work or performance at work severely limited. Housewives and old people able to do light housework only, but able to go out shopping
3 Not in 4 but severe social disability and/or slight impairment of performance at work. Able to do all housework except very heavy tasks
2 Not in 3 but slight social disability
1 No disability

Source: From Rosser & Kind (1978).

consensus view disagreed with the therapists' ratings. Inter-rater reliability among therapists was high ($r = 0.84$).

Disability

The disability scale from the *Charing Cross Health Index* (Rosser & Kind, 1978) was used to assess the overall level of psychosocial functioning of each person (see Table 9.7). This scale has been validated for use to assess disability across a wide range of health problems and covers the full range of potential disability. Of course, most disability associated with mental disorders does not involve severely constricted mobility, but a few cases of severe dystonic side effects of drugs and suicide attempts may result in these levels of impairment. The straightforward nature of the scale made up for inadequacies in terms of specificity of psychosocial deficits. Inter-rater reliability was acceptable ($r = 0.75$).

Handicap

Handicap refers to lost opportunities that are associated with disabilities, such as lack of jobs, friends, housing, finances, etc. People may be capable of working or socialising, but problems such as a lack of provision of resources in the community, or discriminatory practices prevent them from performing the social roles of

Table 9.8. *Global Carer/*
Household Stress Scale

---

0 No stress or carer burden
1 Mild stress or carer burden
2 Moderate stress or carer
burden
3 Severe stress or carer burden

Source: From Falloon (1985).

which they are capable. The complex interaction between ability and social factors makes handicap extraordinarily difficult to measure. To date we have not devised a method that could be applied across all cases.

However, the burden of caring for a person with a mental disorder may be considered a measure of handicap for the informal carers. We employed a modified version of the *Global Carer/ Household Stress Rating (CSR)* from the Social Behaviour Assessment Schedule (Platt et al, 1980) to assess the level that the key carer was disadvantaged on account of his or her care role towards the patient. This four-point global rating (see Table 9.8) was made after review of carers' stresses, lifestyle and personal goals and reflected the disruption in their lives that was directly associated with the patient's mental disorder. Where stress was associated with family, marital or other intimate relationship conflicts, the scale was employed to estimate the levels of *household stress*. Acceptable inter-rater reliability was again achieved between therapists ($r = 0.76$).

Schedule for assessment

These ratings were made at the time a case was first assessed, then at monthly intervals for three months and every three months subsequently. Independent ratings were conducted on a random sample of cases by the evaluation officer employed by the service. This provided an independent audit of case management, as well as reliability check for therapists. Discrepancies in ratings or concerns about the quality of the clinical management were discussed in a constructive manner at the weekly team review meetings.

Cost analysis

This was based upon a continuous record of all professional services provided for each case. This included all time spent in face-to-face contact with patients or carers, telephone consultation, case review and supervision, as well as all services provided by the primary care, hospital, social services, police services, and benefit payments. Monetary benefits accruing from paid employment as well as contributions to the community in the form of voluntary employment were recorded, as well as any loss of earnings of patients or carers, or additional expenditure that was a direct or indirect result of the mental disorder. These data enabled the total costs of integrated care to be estimated.

Preliminary findings

The detailed findings of the cost-effectiveness analysis of the Buckingham Project will be presented in a series of scientific reports and are not presented here. However, the main clinical findings relevant to service development will be summarised in terms of the critical components of the service.

Early intervention

It was evident that the incidence of major mental disorders appeared considerably lower than the levels found in community surveys (see Table 9.2 and Figures 9.1 & 9.2). These levels of detection of mental disorders remained low when compared with data from surveys of hospital admissions (Shepherd et al, 1989; Der et al, 1990; Dilling & Weyrerer, 1984; Goldberg & Huxley, 1980; Myers et al, 1984) – a 10-fold reduction in expected levels of schizophrenic and major affective disorders (Falloon, 1992; Falloon et al, 1992).

While some of this reduction may have been due to conservative diagnostic criteria, the reductions were remarkable and readily noted by clinicians. Family practitioners commented on the substantial reductions they saw in severely impaired new cases, and mental health therapists complained that their skills at managing major episodes of mental disorders were not being exercised. A search of surrounding mental hospitals found no new cases who had sought treatment from neighbouring services whilst registered

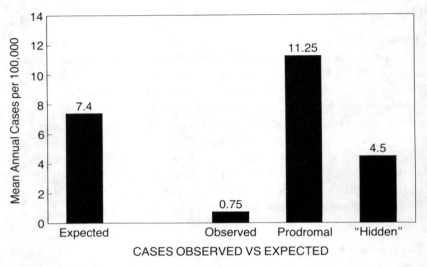

Figure 9.1. The observed versus expected incidence of schizophrenia over a 4-year period.

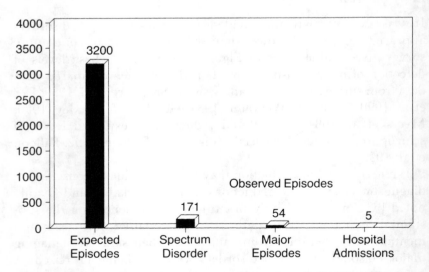

Figure 9.2. The annual prevalence of depressive disorders per 100,000 adults aged between 18 and 65 years.

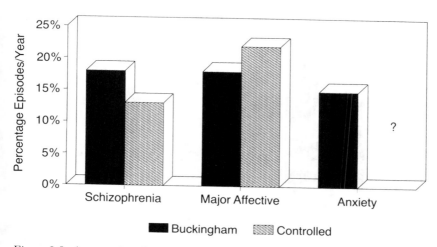

Figure 9.3. A comparison between the percentage of patients experiencing recurrent major episodes of mental disorders in an integrated mental health service and controlled clinical studies of prophylactic intervention strategies.

with local family practices (Andrews, 1990). Thus, it was probable that the early intervention with cases in the early phases of major mental disorders using optimal combinations of biomedical and psychosocial strategies contributed to a lowering of the rate of major episodes of some mental disorders.

A similar reduction was observed in the frequency of recurrent episodes in people who had established disorders (Figure 9.3). This reduction was very similar to that observed in controlled outcome studies that employed the methods we adapted to clinical practice (Falloon & Shanahan, 1990; Teasdale, 1988). Thus, it was evident that these state-of-the-art methods could be applied in everyday mental health service practice with similar benefits.

It was noted that almost no studies of anxiety disorders reported remission and recovery rates (O'Sullivan & Marks, 1989). Furthermore, it was evident that high levels of disability and handicap were associated with persisting impairment in many cases of serious anxiety disorders, even after extensive treatment with optimal cognitive-behavioural and targeted drug strategies. Substantial reductions in target symptoms were usually obtained, but full remissions were rare, particularly in long-term cases, where disability was often higher than in schizophrenic and affective disorders.

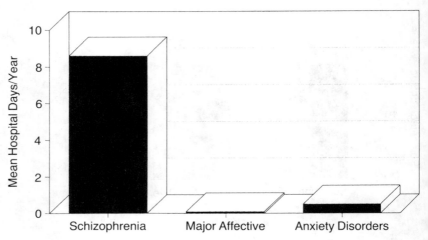

Figure 9.4. Mental hospital inpatient utilisation by long-term patients.

Thus, the community-based perspective of mental disorders tended to reverse that of the hospital-based view that neurotic disorders are less disabling than the functional psychoses and that greater resources should be allocated to the long-term rehabilitation of the latter.

Intensive treatment

The success of early intervention strategies in reducing the number of major episodes of mental disorders contributed to a reduction in the need for intensive treatment, either at home or in hospital (Figure 9.4). On almost no occasion did the provision of 24-hour intensive treatment exceed a rate of five cases per 100,000 and the provision of hospital-based care of major episodes averaged one bed per 100,000. This tended to replicate the findings of similar studies of community-based alternatives to hospital (Stein and Test, 1980; Fenton et al, 1980; Hoult et al, 1983; Hoult, 1986). However, many cases received intensive care that was equivalent to that provided in day hospital units. This could amount to several therapy sessions a week from the key therapist or from several members of the multidisciplinary team. The aim was always to provide the optimal amount of the optimal therapy – no more or no less than was deemed necessary to expedite recovery.

Long-term management

Rehabilitation was initiated at the onset of intervention with efforts to maintain, and wherever possible, to extend social role functioning in the community, this was continued until all impairment, disability and handicap associated with the mental disorder had been eliminated. Any increase in the effectiveness of early intervention and intensive care might be expected to be reflected in a reduction in the need for long-term management. There was some evidence to support this. In, 1984 the number of cases receiving long-term management was 110 (or 370 per 100,000); by 1987 this number had shrunk to 43 (134 per 100,000). However, at that stage the more stringent criteria for long-term management were introduced to ensure that all cases with residual disabilities continued to receive active rehabilitation, and that transfer from specialised to primary care monitoring was delayed until 24 months after all clinical and social morbidity had remitted. This resulted in an increase in long-term management cases to 72 (216 per 100,000). Each year between 10 and 20 cases are added to the long-term management program (see Table 9.3). In the main, half these cases have recovered from major episodes, and half are established cases who have moved into the area, the population of which is one of the most rapidly growing in Europe. One-sixth of all new cases of mental disorders assessed by the service were immigrants. More than half these cases were experiencing adjustment disorders clearly related to the stress of moving.

However, among the 'new' cases of long-term mental disorders are a few who are still being uncovered in the community, and who have not yet received treatment for long-standing major disorders. The additions to long-term management appear to be balanced by a similar number of cases returning to primary care monitoring, and people moving away from the area. In most instances such a move is associated with constructive efforts to a find improved employment or housing opportunities. Virtually no cases have relocated in order to seek improved mental health services. One case moved to a neighbouring area as a direct result of his mental disorder. Despite considerable efforts to ensure that people transferring from our service are linked to effective services in their new locations, several people have found deficiencies in the management elsewhere, with resulting deterioration in their disorders.

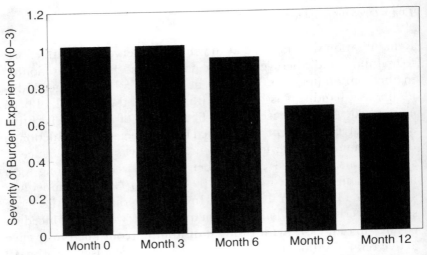

Figure 9.5. The burden experienced by carers during twelve months of integrated long-term care.

Surveys have revealed a continuing trend towards reductions in disability and in the burdens of carers (Figure 9.5). Consistent with our findings in intensive care, we have found that people suffering from the effects of functional psychoses have shown greater improvements in the quality of life of patients and carers than long-term anxiety disorders, particularly obsessive compulsive disorders (Wilkinson et al, 1990).

Economic analysis

The preceding discussion has offered evidence for the effectiveness of an integrated approach to mental health care. The cost of achieving those benefits is of considerable interest to those who may be considering planning such an approach. We have undertaken cost–benefit analyses of both the early intervention and long-term management aspects of the program.

The major costs of a health service are associated with personnel. Figure 9.6 shows that therapeutic activities comprised two-thirds of all the activities of the entire staff, including non-clinical personnel. Figure 9.7 provides a breakdown of key elements of therapeutic input, and shows that the proportion of face-to-face contact between therapist and patients tends to vary according to the type of intervention being delivered. Long-term management cases

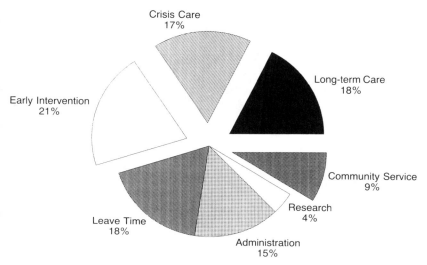

Figure 9.6. A survey of the allocation of staff time.

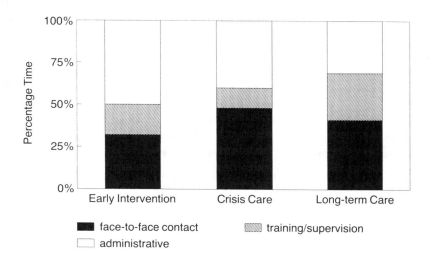

Time calculations include all members of
the service: clinical and administrative

Figure 9.7. The proportion of time clinicians spent in face-to-face contact with patients in an integrated mental health service.

Table 9.9. *Benefits after three months of
integrated care: reduction in impairment,
disability and carer stress*

	Mean change per case	Total for 376 cases
Reduction on scales of:		
Impairment	0.94	355
Disability	0.74	180
Carer/family stress	0.70	262
Number of sessions		
Mental health	4.92	1851
Primary care	1.75	658
Other services	0.10	37
Hospital days		
General hospital		15
Mental hospital		42

received a higher proportion of face-to-face contact, whereas with early intervention cases substantially more service time was spent making records, in case conferences and in supervision and consultation activities. It was pleasing to note that the greatest time in face-to-face contact was spent with long-term cases, and the least with the much more numerous and demanding early intervention cases. Therapist members of the service spent an average of 48% of their time at work in direct patient contact. This included those consulting members of the clinical team (psychiatrists, psychologists, social workers and occupational therapists), who were expected to spend most of their time in indirect supervisory roles. Thus, most of the nursing therapists spent an even higher proportion of their time in face-contact with patients and their carers. The comprehensive cost of one hour of face-to-face contact with the service was estimated as £29.00 (in 1988–98). This included all administrative and overhead costs.

Cost–benefit analyses have been conducted on both short-term and long-term aspects of the integrated service. Table 9.9 summarises the benefits associated with the first three months of treatment in the service, as well as the major therapeutic components provided during that early intervention phase. In this analysis each unit of benefit was considered to represent a reduction of one point on the global scales of impairment (CGI), disability (Charing Cross Health Index), and carer or household stress (CSR). It may be noted that benefits were evenly distributed across the three measures, and that the average benefits to each case totalled 2.6. These benefits were achieved with around seven sessions of professional input, with a small component provided in hospital settings. The cost to patients and their families as a result of time away from work, and additional household costs were minimised by the home-based approach to intensive care, and amounted to a very small cost per case. Similarly, the targeted approach to drug treatment limited the use of drugs for many cases, with only a quarter receiving pharmacotherapy, with relatively few receiving continuous drug treatment throughout the three months. The cost of the clinical management of each case was £218. The cost per unit benefit was estimated at £91, with the direct costs to the mental health budget of £60 per unit benefit.

The benefits associated with integrated care of those cases assessed as having mental disorders were three times greater than those associated with the clinical management of people with psychosocial difficulties. Furthermore, the cost of each unit of benefit was £90 for persons suffering from mental disorders and £148 for those experiencing only psychosocial problems. This finding might be considered a disincentive for assessment and treatment of cases who are not deemed to have a mental disorder. However, these data are somewhat distorted by the fact that psychosocial cases were not able to show any benefits on the clinical assessment. One-quarter of these cases were rated as within normal limits on each of the three scales at the initial assessment and consequently could not demonstrate any benefits at all from the intervention. Although most of these cases received no more than brief stress management counselling, it is important to clarify whether this was an appropriate use of health care resources. The question as to whether these efforts were associated with the low rates of inception of major mental disorders cannot be answered. At present there can be no justification for diverting precious mental health resources away from the clinical care of people with mental disorders or their prodromal states on the grounds that stress management may prevent the development of initial episodes of these conditions.

A similar economic analysis of the efficiency of long term management of 40 cases showed that over a one-year period they had

achieved an average of one unit of clinical, social or family benefit
from their baseline states. This benefit was achieved at a cost of
£1500 to the integrated primary care and mental health services. It
was of interest to note that these long-term cases utilised minimal
specialised rehabilitation services, such as day care, home help,
sheltered work, etc. The carer-based problem-solving approach
enabled them to access a wide range of rehabilitation resources
within the community, with relatively few of their needs being unmet
in this manner. Further, it was observed that rather than place
added burdens on informal carers this home-based approach tended
to relieve them of some of their stress (see Figure 9.5).

Adaptability

There are no data to suggest that an integrated service provides
greater adaptability than a hospital-based community service. However, it will be evident that highly flexible deployment of resources is
feasible with such a model. This is particularly crucial in the
deployment of intensive treatment and long-term management
resources. Intensive management can be provided wherever and
whenever it is required providing sufficient staff are available to
deliver the treatment. Carers and patients themselves are co-opted
as members of the therapy team, enabling professionals to devote
their efforts to targeted specialised interventions, rather than general
support. The number of 'beds' served at any time will more closely
approximate the current needs of the community rather than the
constraints of the more rigid capacity of an institution. When the
need for intensive management of crises is minimal resources can be
readily switched to intensive rehabilitation efforts with the most
disabled cases.

Such adaptability needs excellent team coordination to ensure
that priority is given to the areas of greatest need, and mobilise
resources to target a specific crisis with maximal efficiency. Figure
9.7 suggests that a balance between the various phases of case
management can be achieved. At times of reduced staffing the
balance between needs and resources may be compromised
occasionally. However, the expectation that all members of the
service may be called upon to carry out a range of interventions,

including crisis nursing management, enables most needs to be met in a near optimal fashion.

As provision of management of the mentally disordered has shifted from the traditional hospital-based emphasis on functional psychoses to anxiety and adjustment disorders, there has been a tendency for some family practitioners to request assistance for increasing numbers of people distressed by emotional and social crises. We have resisted the temptation to develop specific services within our service for such cases and have lobbied for improved social services, including counselling services to meet this need. Several of our staff have volunteered their services to assist in the development of such services and in the training of counsellors. However, it has been understood that such voluntary service may only be undertaken during work hours when all the needs of the mentally disordered people and their carers have been met. Such service must be curtailed immediately a crisis arises.

Indices of adaptability are difficult to devise. However, it is crucial that efforts are made to develop such measures, so that service development can be targeted to the changing needs of the community.

References

Andrews G. (1990) England: An innovative community psychiatric service. *Lancet*, **i**, 1087–1088.

Birch C. (1990) Client satisfaction. Research report for English Nursing Board course #811 (unpublished).

Cardin V., McGill C.W. & Falloon I.R.H. (1985) An economic analysis: costs, benefits and effectiveness. In I.R.H. Falloon (Ed.) *Family management of schizophrenia*. Johns Hopkins University Press, Baltimore.

Chen A. (1991) Noncompliance in community psychiatry: a review of clinical interventions. *Hospital & Community Psychiatry*, **42**, 282–286.

Clark I. (1989) Letter. *Lancet*.

Der G., Gupta G. & Murray R.M. (1990) Is schizophrenia disappearing? *Lancet*, **335**, 513–516.

Dilling H. & Weyrerer S. (1984) Prevalence of mental disorders in the small town rural region of Traunstein (Upper Bavaria). *Acta Psychiatrica Scandinavica*, **69**, 60–79.

Falloon I.R.H. (1992) Early intervention for first episodes of schizophrenia. *Psychiatry*, **55**, 4–15.

Falloon I.R.H. (1985) *Family management of schizophrenia.* Johns Hopkins University Press, Baltimore.

Falloon I.R.H. & Shanahan W.J. (1990) Community management of schizophrenia. *British Journal of Hospital Medicine,* **43**, 62–66.

Falloon I.R.H., Shanahan W. & Laporta M. (1992) Prevention of major depressive episodes: early intervention with family-based stress management. *Journal of Mental Health,* **1**, 53–60.

Falloon I.R.H. & Talbot R.E. (1982) The goals of day treatment. *Journal of Nervous and Mental Disease,* **170**, 279–85.

Fenton F.R., Tessier L., Struening E.L., Smith F.A. & Benoit C. (1982) *Home and hospital psychiatric treatment.* Croom Helm, London.

Goldberg D. & Blackwell B.(1970) Psychiatric illness in general practice: a detailed study using a new method of case identification. *British Medical Journal,* **ii**, 439–443.

Goldberg D.P. & Huxley P. (1980) *Mental illness in the community: The pathway to psychiatric care.* Tavistock, London.

Guy W. (1976) *E.C.D.E.U. assessment manual for psychopharmacology.* U.S. Department of Health, Education and Welfare, Washington, D.C.

Hoult J. (1986) Community care for the acutely mentally ill. *British Journal of Psychiatry,* **149**, 137–144.

Hoult J., Reynolds I., Charbonneau-Powis M., Weekes P. & Briggs J. (1983) Psychiatric hospital versus community treatment: Results of a randomised trial. *Australian & New Zealand Journal of Psychiatry,* **17**, 160–167.

Kluger M.P. & Karras A. (1983) Strategies for reducing initial appointments in a community mental health center. *Community Mental Health Journal,* **19**, 137–143.

Lee A.S. & Murray R.M. (1988) The long-term outcome of Maudsley depressives. *British Journal of Psychiatry,* **153**, 741–751.

Myers J.K., Weissman M.M., Tischler G.L., Leaf P.J., Orvascel H., Anthony J.C., Boyd J.H., Burke J.D., Kramer M. & Stoltzman R. (1984) Six-month prevalence of psychiatric disorders in three communities:, 1980 to, 1982. *Archives of General Psychiatry,* **41**, 959–967.

Newman S.C., Shrout P.E. & Bland R.C. (1990) The efficiency of two-phase designs in prevalence surveys of mental disorders. *Psychological Medicine,* **20**, 183–194.

O'Sullivan G. & Marks I. (1991) Long-term follow-up of agoraphobia, panic and obsessive-compulsive disorders. In R Noyes (Ed.) *Handbook of anxiety,* Vol. 4. Elsevier, Amsterdam.

Platt S., Weyman A., Hirsch S. & Hewett S. (1980) The social behaviour assessment schedule (SBAS): Rationale, contents, scoring and reliability of a new intervention schedule. *Social Psychiatry,* **15**, 43–55.

Renvoize E. & Clayden D. (1990) Can suicide rate be used as a performance indicator in mental illness? *Health Trends,* **12**, 16–19.

Rosser R.M. & Kind P. (1978) A scale of valuations of states of illness: Is there a social consensus? *International Journal of Epidemiology*, **7**, 347–358.

Shepherd M., Watt D., Falloon I. & Smeeton N. (1989) *The natural history of schizophrenia: a five-year follow-up study of outcome and prediction in a representative sample of schizophrenics*. Psychological Medicine Monograph 16, Cambridge University Press, Cambridge.

Stein L.I. & Test M.A. (1980) An alternative to mental hospital treatment: I. Conceptual model, treatment program, and clinical evaluation. *Archives of General Psychiatry*, **37**, 392–399.

Strathdee G., King M.B., Araya R. & Lewis S.A. (1990) A standardized assessment of patients referred to primary care and hospital psychiatric clinics. *Psychological Medicine*, **20**, 219–224

Taylor S.J. (1989) A comparison of mental health services. (Three outpatient clinics in the Oxford Health Region). Dissertation completed as part of BSc. degree, Oxford Polytechnic.

Teasdale J. (1988) Cognitive therapy for depression: the state of the art. Paper presented at the World Congress of Behaviour Therapy, Edinburgh, September 8, 1988.

Tyrer P. (1984) Psychiatric clinics in general practice: an extension of community care. *British Journal of Psychiatry*, **145**, 9–14.

Wilkinson G., Croft-Jeffreys C., Krekorian H., McLees S. & Falloon I.R.H. (1990) QALYS in psychiatric care? *Psychiatric Bulletin*, **14**, 582–585.

10
Conclusions and future directions

Integrated care aims to provide the optimal clinical management for all people who experience mental disorders in a defined community. This includes detecting disorders at the earliest possible stage, providing intensive biomedical and psychosocial interventions to minimise impairment, disability and handicaps associated with the disorder, including the stress associated with caring for sufferers; and ensuring that future episodes are prevented wherever possible. There is tentative evidence to suggest that such an approach is feasible and that the results are similar to those found in controlled clinical trials. Moreover, both consumers and providers appear pleased with the integrated approach that ensures that treatment is provided in and around the home, in a manner that attempts to address the expressed personal needs of individuals and their carers, and involves a full range of community resources, particularly those provided by the primary health care services.

With such a service, not only are mental hospital provisions minimal, but specialised day hospitals and outpatient clinics are seldom needed. Instead the focus is on the provision of therapeutic interventions in the natural environment, with therapists' skill and training the major resource required to develop and maintain a quality service. The therapeutic interventions that are employed are chosen on the basis of efficacy and efficiency, and care is taken to ensure that all mental health professionals are trained to deploy these cost-effective clinical management strategies in a highly competent manner. In addition to extensive and continual training of specialist professionals in the latest advances in intervention strategies, efforts have been made to provide specific training for members of the primary care services, including community nurses and family practitioners. This latter training focusses on the recognition of the early stages of mental disorders, and targeted pharmacotherapy.

The role of informal carers, both families and friends, is considered crucial to the integrated care approach. Assessment of their strengths and weaknesses as key members of the care team is followed by education and training to assist them to provide the optimal support for the people for whom they are caring in their own homes. Integrated management similarly attempts to assist those people who are suffering from mental disorders to become active participants in their own care. Self-help is encouraged, and specific training is provided in a wide range of drug and psychosocial strategies that are targeted to specific symptoms, such as anxiety, depression and mania, sleep and appetite disturbances, hallucinations and delusions, aggressive and suicidal behaviours. Combinations of low dose drug with psychosocial stress management strategies are utilised as long-term prophylaxis against recurrent episodes of major mental disorders.

In addition to efforts to minimise clinical morbidity, integrated care places considerable emphasis on the restoration of a full range of functioning through continued rehabilitation procedures. These include specific training in occupational, interpersonal and recreational skills, as well as strategies to ensure that full access is provided to all facilities and resources available in the community. Every person, no matter how severe their disabilities, is expected to be able to lead a full and satisfying life in the community.

Integration occurs at several different levels – between specialist, primary and informal carers; between biomedical, psychological and social management; between early intervention, intensive crisis care, and extensive long-term rehabilitation. Whereas such an approach requires little adjustment for primary and informal care systems, who tend to work in a similar manner for most cases, this method is a major departure from the traditionally hospital-based specialist services. However, our experience has shown that establishing teams of mental health professionals who are able to integrate fully with their primary care colleagues, and above all within the social environments of patients and their carers, can be achieved with relatively little difficulty.

Among the minor difficulties that have been encountered have been the need for flexible staffing to permit professionals to provide the different levels of care – early intervention, intensive care and long-term care – often all three levels in the same day. Similar flexibility has been needed to ensure that the range of specialist resources are available when needed with minimal delays. Such flexibility is relatively easy to arrange among committed clinicians, but provokes administrative resistance within public sector facilities. The wide changes in the prevalence of health problems that have been noted with the changing seasons are seldom matched by changes in staffing resources. We have noted that intensive care for major mental disorders is in greatest demand during the spring and autumn months and least during winter and summer. A constant provision of professional resources means that services are stretched at certain times and under-utilised at others. This ebb and flow is consistent, and can be moderated by encouraging leave to be taken during the slack periods, taking steps to maximise the health of staff so that they are at less risk of succumbing to health problems themselves, and to ensure that any spare capacity is readily used to provide extensive rehabilitation of disabled persons.

A few family practitioners have complained that the integrated approach tends to reduce the choice of patients to be referred to specific professionals or clinics. On occasions requests have been made for therapists of a specific sex, or an inefficient therapeutic strategy not currently provided by the service. The response to such requests has been to educate the practitioner concerned about evidence for the efficacy of the requested management and to outline the most effective strategies for resolving the presenting problems of the case concerned. The resulting *informed choice* has almost always concurred with the management advocated by the mental health therapists.

Initially family practitioners expressed concern that psychiatric assessments could only be conducted by qualified psychiatrists, and were reluctant to consult with non-medical colleagues. However, when they realised that all members of the integrated service had been trained to administer psychiatric assessments to the same degree of reliability as experienced psychiatrists, they were reassured. Although all mental health professionals can be trained to conduct reliable mental status assessments and background information, the clinical management of all people experiencing episodes of major mental disorders should remain under the close supervision of the team psychiatrists at all times, in a manner similar to that pertaining in inpatient units. The integrated approach places the main emphasis of development of mental health care services on the training of all members of the clinical team, so that every person in the community that is being served is able to receive the optimal assessment and treatment strategies for any mental disorder that they should have the misfortune to experience.

In addition to the training and clinical supervision provided by psychiatrists, similar roles should be adopted by psychologists, nurses, social workers and occupational therapists when their less specialised colleagues conduct clinical procedures that are derived from their specialty. Such demarcation may prevent excessive blurring of professional expertise that is considered a threat by many professions and often hampers attempts at close teamwork.

It was apparent that the careful application of the most recent developments in mental health care contributed to recovery from many potentially disabling mental disorders, and assisted in minimising the handicaps of those suffering from persisting disabilities. Unfortunately recovery from serious mental disorders was not universal, and it was apparent that some disorders tended to respond better than others. Furthermore this differential response to clinical management contrasted to that noted from a hospital-based perspective. Episodes of depression, schizophrenia, mania and panic tended to respond readily and usually completely to state-of-the-art interventions, whilst obsessive-compulsive and anxiety disorders showed much lower rates of clinical or social recovery. Substantial changes on rating scales in these latter disorders were similar to those found in research studies, but often left residual symptoms that were associated with continued disability. For example, one woman reduced her time spent on daily rituals by 60%, but still spent four hours checking and washing, and was unable to extend her social function to any worthwhile extent. It became evident that these disorders which present in less dramatic fashion are readily forgotten by primary care services and hospital-based services alike. However, it seems crucial that further efforts, both in developing more effective clinical intervention strategies, and in rehabilitation, should focus on these disorders, which are all too often dismissed as trivial. It was apparent that when these disorders were treated at an early stage in their development that the response tended to be much better. The major lifestyle changes of both patients and their carers that often to occur as attempts to accommodate long-term disabilities tend to perpetuate the impairments and make effective clinical intervention a much more complex process. For this reason it appears important that all mental disorders are detected and treated at the earliest possible stage. Refinements in detection procedures must involve primary care services as well as improved community understanding about mental health care. The integrated care approach provides considerable scope for potential developments in these important areas.

A final problem that was observed concerned the migration of established cases of mental disorders. It was notable that a disproportionate number of the people who experienced major episodes of mental disorders had recently moved into the area. Few of these cases had informed their family practitioners of their previous episodes of mental disorders until they presented with a major episode. Attempts were made to screen all cases registering with the family practices in the area. However, many people were afraid to disclose a history of mental disorder. Several reported that they suspected that such disclosure had led to rejection by family practices in the past. It seems crucial that people who are vulnerable to stress-related disorders are carefully monitored at times of major stress, and few stresses are as great as those associated with relocation. We devised a procedure whereby people leaving the area sought out a new family practitioner before they moved and that reports were provided, both written, and on occasions where a high risk of a recurrent episode was likely, through telephone conversations. Patients and their carers were given copies of the written reports in case they had to seek emergency assistance when the new practitioner was unavailable. This procedure appeared to work extremely well. In addition, patients and their carers received extensive training in stress management procedures to prepare for the stresses they anticipated throughout the relocation period.

The future prospects of providing effective and efficient mental health care that meets the needs of communities appear enhanced by the development of the integrated approach. Accessibility, acceptability, accountability and adaptability all seem improved when compared with the traditional hospital-based approach to service delivery. While current clinical management appears highly effective, particularly when applied in a comprehensive manner in the early phases of major disorders, limitations in treatment efficacy leave a small proportion of cases with persisting disability. It is hoped that future innovation in treatment methods combined with more efficient case detection and service delivery will provide further advances in the years to come.

Appendixes. Semi-structured assessments used in an integrated mental health service

Appendix 1   **Community health record**

Name ................................D.O.B. ....

Address ....

Tel ....Marital Status ....

GP ....Date referred ....

Presenting problems   Duration

1._____   _____

2._____   _____

3._____   _____

Reason(s) for referral

1._____

2._____

3._____

Current management

1._____

2._____

3._____

Other services (Health Visitor, District Nurse, Midwife,

Social Worker, etc.) ....

Therapist ....Date seen ....

History of problems: _____

_____

_____

_____

_____

_____

Past history (Medical and mental health): _____

_____

_____

_____

Family history: _____

_____

_____

_____

Social history. Developmental: _____

_____

_____

_____

Occupational: _____

_____

Financial: _____

Housing: _____

Diagnosis: 1 _____

(DSM-IIIR, Axis I)

2 _____

Target problems/goals

1 _____

2 _____

Management plans:

1 _____

2 _____

3 _____

4 _____

5 _____

Progress notes:

_____

_____

_____

_____

_____

_____

_____

_____

_____

_____

_____

_____

_____

_____

_____

_____

Appendix 2   **Mental health assessment**

CLIENT NO. |...|...|...|...| IS THIS A NEW REFERRAL?   YES/NO

SURNAME: _____

FIRST NAME: _____

DATE OF BIRTH: |...|...|...| SEX: MALE/FEMALE

ADDRESS _____

_____

_____

TEL NO. HOME: _____   WORK: _____

DATE REFERRED: _____

DATE SEEN: _____

GP: _____

OTHER CONTACT AGENCY INVOLVED (Please specify): _____

_____

_____

ASSESSED BY: _____

KEY WORKER: _____

DATE OF TRANSFER TO MENTAL HEALTH FOLLOW-UP: _____

DATE OF TRANSFER TO GP FOLLOW-UP: _____

HAS PERSON COOPERATED WITH

CLINICAL MANAGEMENT? .... FULLY/PARTLY/NOT

AT ALL

                                         NAME:

                                A

FAMILY MEMBER: |...|...|...|...|...| _____

                                B

FAMILY MEMBER: |...|...|...|...|...| _____

                                C

FAMILY MEMBER: |...|...|...|...|...| _____

                                D

FAMILY MEMBER: |...|...|...|...|...| _____

MARITAL STATUS (circle code):
 1 Presently married
 2 Sustained conjugal relationship/living permanently
    with someone
 3 Widowed
 4 Divorced
 5 Separated
 6 Never married

HOUSEHOLD DURING PAST 3 MONTHS (circle members):
Spouse/Partner   Mother   Father
Children (No.) |...| Siblings (No.) |...|
Other relatives (No.) |...| Non-relatives (No.) |...|
COMMENTS _____

FAMILY TYPE (circle code):
 1 Parental or lineal (person referred does not carry major financial
    responsibility for the home; it is either the home of family of
    origin/or of children)
 2 Conjugal/marital (person or spouse/partner carried major
    responsibility for the home; the household may include parents or
    children)
 3 Alone (home may be shared with others not related to person, or may
    live in unsupervised lodgings, dormitory, etc. but has financial
    responsibility)
 4 Collateral (home is not the responsibility of person, parents or
    children, but of sibling, aunt or some other non-linear relative)
 5 Structured environment (e.g., supervised hostel, halfway house,
    board and care, co-operative apartment, other supervised or
    supportive residences)

HIGHEST LEVEL OF EDUCATION (circle code):
 1 University degree
 2 Sixth form School/College (A levels)
 3 Secondary School with O levels, GCSEs, CSEs
 4 Secondary School without examinations
 5 No Secondary School

OCCUPATIONAL STATUS:
Employed/student/housewife at present: YES/NO
What is the present job? _____
Number of months he/she has been working in the past 24
months: |...|...|
If unemployed, is person able to work at usual job?   YES/NO
Past occupations (and duration): _____
_____
_____

MEDICAL HISTORY

(A) Please state main medical complaints in past, including operations (if none, please state)

_____

(B) Please list any present medical complaints and drug treatment (if none, please state)

_____

PAST MENTAL HEALTH

Has person received mental health care before?   YES/NO

AGE	DIAGNOSIS	TREATMENTS	DURATION	OUTCOME
___	_____	_____	_____	_____
___	_____	_____	_____	_____

Has person been admitted to hospital for mental health care?
YES/NO
How many times? _____
Total duration of hospital care: _____ months.
Has person received medication for treatment of mental
disorder?   YES/NO
What medications? (dose & duration)

_____

FAMILY HISTORY

Have any of the following relatives had a history of
psychiatric treatment?
code 0 – if there is no history of illness at all
      1 – if had been ill and treated by GP
      2 – if had been ill and treated by mental health service
            SPECIfY NATURE OF DISORDER

Father _____ |...|
Mother _____ |...|
Children _____ |...| |...| |...|
Siblings _____ |...| |...| |...|

VULNERABILITY—STRESS CHECKLIST

Check boxes (X) to indicate vulnerability—stress factors that are present in this case. Where unknown or unsure place a ? in the box. Where absent place (0) in the box.

1. Previous episode(s) of depressive symptoms. ☐
2. Previous episode(s) of schizophrenic symptoms. ☐
3. Previous episode(s) of manic symptoms. ☐
4. Loss of mother before 11 years of age. ☐
5. Lack of social competence in adolescence. ☐
6. 2 or more preschool children at home. ☐
7. Unemployed for 12 months (or more) out of last 24 months. ☐
8. Absence of confiding, close relationship. ☐
9. Persistent family/marital tension. ☐
10. Major life event in the past year (bereavement, divorce, relocation, major illness, job loss, etc). ☐
11. Persistent major life stress (e.g. financial, housing, chronic illness). ☐
12. Persisting hopelessness about ability to resolve problems. ☐
13. Long-term (6 months) minor tranquilliser/ antidepressant use. ☐
14. Caffeine abuse (more than 5 cups tea or coffee or cola). ☐
15. Tobacco smoking. ☐
16. Alcohol or drug abuse (used as coping strategy). ☐

COMMENTS: _____
_____
_____

ALCOHOL & DRUG HISTORY

(A)   Does person drink alcohol?   YES/NO
      <u>IF</u> YES rate how much he/she drinks per week (one unit of
      alcohol equals standard glass of wine/half a pint of beer
      or lager/standard measure of spirit)
      No. of Units [|]

(B)   Does patient abuse drugs at present time? (not
      prescribed by medical profession)   YES/NO

<u>IF</u> YES specify drug/s used & frequency _____

Family history of substance abuse: YES/NO
(whom and what) _____

PROBLEM ANALYSIS

PROBLEM 1 : _____
_____
_____

BRIEF HISTORY OF PROBLEM : _____
_____
_____

ANTECEDENTS : _____
_____
_____

CONSEQUENCES : _____
_____
_____

FREQUENCY/INTENSITY : _____
MODIFYING FACTORS (What makes problem better?) : _____
_____
_____

(What makes problem worse?) : _____
_____
_____

GAINS/LOSSES FROM RESOLUTION : _____
_____
_____

WHO DO YOU SOLVE PROBLEMS WITH : _____
CURRENT PROBLEM-SOLVING EFFORTS : _____
_____
_____
_____

ASSETS/DEFICITS IN PROBLEM RESOLUTION : _____
_____
_____
_____
_____

PROBLEM 2: _____

_____

BRIEF HISTORY OF PROBLEM: _____

_____

ANTECEDENTS: _____

_____

CONSEQUENCES: _____

_____

FREQUENCY/INTENSITY: _____
MODIFYING FACTORS (What makes problem better?): ____

_____

(What makes problem worse?): _____

_____

GAINS/LOSSES FROM RESOLUTION: _____

_____

WHO DO YOU SOLVE PROBLEMS WITH: _____
CURRENT PROBLEM-SOLVING EFFORTS: _____

_____

_____

ASSETS/DEFICITS IN PROBLEM RESOLUTION: ____

_____

_____

_____

REINFORCEMENT SURVEY

(Note the activities, people, places and material objects
that person spends most time involved with.)

ACTIVITIES:
Current   1. _____
             2. _____
             3. _____
Preferred   1. _____
             2. _____
             3. _____

PERSONS:
Current   1. _____
             2. _____
             3. _____
Preferred   1. _____
             2. _____
             3. _____

PLACES:
Current   1. _____
             2. _____
             3. _____
Preferred   1. _____
             2. _____
             3. _____

THINGS:
Current   1. _____
             2. _____
             3. _____
Preferred   1. _____
             2. _____
             3. _____

AVERSIVE PEOPLE, PLACES, THINGS AND ACTIVITIES: _____

POTENTIAL REINFORCERS FOR THERAPY (List all readily
available reinforcers that might assist in therapeutic
management, including removal of aversive reinforcers): ____
_____
_____

CURRENT LIFE GOALS

SUBJECT'S FUNCTIONAL GOALS RELEVANT TO INDIVIDUAL AND FAMILY NEEDS. (If your problem were resolved, what would you like to achieve in your life in the next 6 months? Note: realistic goals that would make a significant long-term impact on quality of life.)

GOAL: _____

_____

_____

STEPS ALREADY ACHIEVED: _____

_____

_____

PROBLEMS ANTICIPATED IN ACHIEVING GOAL: _____

_____

_____

ENVIRONMENTAL SUPPORT VS. CONFLICT IN ACHIEVING GOAL: _____

_____

_____

GOAL: _____

_____

STEPS ALREADY ACHIEVED: _____

_____

_____

PROBLEMS ANTICIPATED IN ACHIEVING GOAL: _____

_____

_____

ENVIRONMENTAL SUPPORT VS CONFLICT IN ACHIEVING GOAL: _____

_____

_____

_____

_____

PROBLEM MANAGEMENT PLAN

PROBLEM 1 : _____

HOW IS PROBLEM TO BE MEASURED : _____
_____

WHAT IS THE GOAL OF INTERVENTION : _____
_____

WHAT IS THE BASELINE? _____
_____

WHAT ARE THE METHODS OF INTERVENTION? _____
_____
_____
_____
_____
_____
_____
_____
_____

PROBLEM 2 : _____

HOW IS PROBLEM TO BE MEASURED : _____
_____

WHAT IS THE GOAL OF INTERVENTION : _____
_____

WHAT IS THE BASELINE? _____
_____

WHAT ARE THE METHODS OF INTERVENTION? _____
_____
_____
_____
_____
_____
_____
_____

THERAPIST RATINGS OF CURRENT MENTAL DISORDER
DIAGNOSIS (DSM-IIIR)

	BASELINE	TRANSFER TO GP
AXIS I		
AXIS II		
AXIS III		

PROBLEM

1.
2.

PROBLEM SEVERITY (RATE 0–8)

WEEKS	0	1	2	3	4	5	6	7	8	9	10	11	12
PROBLEM 1													
PROBLEM 2													

(continued)

MONTHS	4	5	6	7	8	9	10	11	12	18	24	36	48	60
PROBLEM 1														
PROBLEM 2														

GLOBAL ASSESSMENT SCALE (SEVERITY OF MENTAL ILLNESS)

MONTHS	0	1	2	3		6	9	12	18	24	36	48	60
SCORES													

CHARING CROSS HEALTH INDICATOR (DISABILITY)

MONTHS	0	1	2	3		6	9	12	18	24	36	48	60
SCORES													

CARER BURDEN/STRESS

MONTHS	0	1	2	3		6	9	12	18	24	36	48	60
SCORES													

PROGRESS RECORD

PATIENT: _____ B.M.H.S. INDEX NO: _____ THERAPIST: _____

DATE	SESSION NO.	TYPE	TARGET PROBLEM(S)	TARGET RATING	SESSION DETAILS	COMMENTS, HOMEWORK, SIGNIFICANT EVENTS	TOTAL HOURS

TYPE OF SESSION:
Clinic attendance (C); Domiciliary visit (D); Supervised Excursion, e.g. public places (E); Telephone (T)

LIFE CHART

Name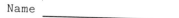

TARGET PROBLEM RATING

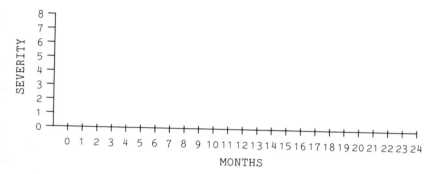

SOCIAL FUNCTIONING

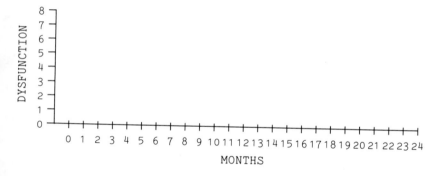

FAMILY BURDEN/STRESS

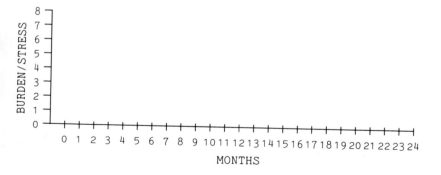

Appendix 3 Long-term case management: Quarterly review

Name of patient .... Name of carer ....
Name of therapist ....
Date assessment due .... Date completed ....

This questionnaire is to be completed at three-month intervals by the therapist of every patient who initially had an Axis I DSM-IIIR diagnosis and meets at least one of the following criteria:
1. has required continuous treatment for illness or disability for at least 12 months
2. has had a previous episode of an Axis I disorder
3. has shown prodromal features of a schizophrenic disorder
4. has vulnerability factors that suggest he/she may develop serious disability from a mental disorder in the future.

Assessments may be discontinued in some cases who remain free of symptoms, warning signs or disability for 24 consecutive months.

A: COMMUNITY TENURE

How much time has patient spent living in the following places during the past 3 months (in weeks)? Specify any changes and details:

(1) Home   [   ] ....
(2) General hospital [   ] ....
(3) Mental hospital [   ] ....
(4) Residential care [   ] ....
(5) Prison, etc.   [   ] ....
(6) Other   [   ] ....
      (include holidays, weekends away, etc.)

Reasons for admissions to institutional care
(code 1 = yes; more than one code may be used)

		Mental Hosp	General Hosp	Resident Care	Prison
1	Clinical exacerbation	[ ]	[ ]	[ ]	[ ]
2	Behaviour disorder	[ ]	[ ]	[ ]	[ ]
3	Family reasons	[ ]	[ ]	[ ]	[ ]
4	Social reasons	[ ]	[ ]	[ ]	[ ]
5	Legal reasons	[ ]	[ ]	[ ]	[ ]
6	Mental Health Act	[ ]	[ ]	[ ]	[ ]
7	Clinical investigation	[ ]	[ ]	[ ]	[ ]
8	Physical disorder	[ ]	[ ]	[ ]	[ ]

B: WORK ACTIVITY

Patient's employment status in last 3 months (include work as housewife, student, sheltered work/volunteer; exclude time in hospital):

(code)

4 .... employed continuously
3 .... employed more than half the time, but less than continuously
2 .... employed part-time or full time about half of the time in the past 3 months
1 .... employed less than half of the time in the past 3 months
0 .... no useful work
8 .... retired

Total number of weeks employed during past 3 months ($= 13$ weeks): [   ]

C: CHARING CROSS HEALTH INDICATOR AND PROFILE

Disability Scale

Code the appropriate categories to demonstrate the state of the patient <u>NOW.</u>

8   Unconscious.
7   Not in 8 but confined to bed.
6   Not in 7 but confined to wheelchair or chair or able to move around in the home only with support from an assistant.
5   Not in 6 but unable to undertake any paid employment. Unable to continue any education. Old people confined to home except for escorted outings and short walks and unable to do shopping. Housewives only able to perform a few simple tasks.
4   Not in 5 but choice of work or performance at work severely limited. Housewives and old people able to do light housework only, but able to go out shopping.
3   Not in 4 but severe social disability and/or slight impairment of performance at work. Able to do all housework except very heavy tasks.
2   Not in 3 but slight social disability.
1   No disability.

D: SEVERITY OF PSYCHOSOCIAL STRESSORS (see DSM-IIIR)

Note ALL stressors, both ambient and life events in past 3 months.

1 NONE
2 MINIMAL   ....
3 MILD   ....
4 MODERATE   ....
5 SEVERE   ....
6 EXTREME   ....
7 CATASTROPHIC ....

E: BURDEN ON CARERS

Invite key carers to assess the level of stress they experience that is related to the patient's disability in the following manner:

Living with someone who suffers from illness can lead to many different kinds of problems. The person's symptoms or general behaviour may cause stress. Going out or inviting friends home may cause concern. Having an emotionally ill person living at home can affect the ability of the other household members to go about their own lives in all manner of ways. In what ways has your family been affected? (note examples). I would like you to give us your opinion of the overall effect that X's mental health problems have had on your home life in the past 3 months.

(1) Code carers global burden   [   ]
    0 none
    1 minimal
    2 moderate
    3 severe

(2) Taking everything into account, how do you feel about continuing to care for X over the next months
    (a) Distress [   ]   (b) Attitude [   ]
    0 none   1 positive ⎫
    1 mild   2 resigned ⎬ about care role
    2 moderate   3 rejecting ⎭
    3 severe

CLINICAL STATUS

Target symptoms (highest level in past 3 months)

1   2   3   4   5   6   7

(doubtful/trivial)   (clearly present)   (very severe)

                                     severity

(1) PSE code [   ] .... [   ]
(2) PSE code [   ] .... [   ]

EARLY WARNING SIGNS (present at any time during past 3 months)

(1) .... [   ] Present = 1
(2) .... [   ] Absent   = 0
(3) .... [   ]

CLINICAL GLOBAL IMPRESSIONS

Highest global rating in the past 3 months

(code from therapist's weekly Clinical Global Impression Scale)

   0 Normal, not at all ill
   1 Borderline mentally ill
   2 Slightly mentally ill   Highest Rating [   ]
   3 Moderately ill
   4 Markedly ill
   5 Severely ill
   6 Among the most extremely ill patients

CURRENT DIAGNOSIS

Diagnosis at this moment (DSM-IIIR; Axis I) _____

(Note: If disorder in full remission code = V71.09)

Comments:

....
....
....
....
....
....
....
....
....
....
....
....
....

CLINICAL MANAGEMENT PLAN FOR NEXT 3 MONTHS

Patient Goals: (1) ....
(2) ....
(3) ....
Carer Goals: (1) ....
(2) ....
(3) ....
Medication: Name   Dose

....
....
....

Other Medical Strategies ....

Psychological Strategies: ....
(incl. OT)

....
....
....

Social Strategies:
....
....

COSTS AND BENEFITS (for past three months)
Costs: Direct)

Hours spent in face-to-face contact in last 3 months, to nearest half-hour
double time if two therapists, etc)

		Home	Clinic	Emergency	
NH Therapy Session:	IND	[ ]	[ ]	[ ]	....
	FAM	[ ]	[ ]	[ ]	....
	GRP	[ ]	[ ]	[ ]	....
	OTHER	[ ]	[ ]	[ ]	....
OT Assessment		[ ]	[ ]	[ ]	
Psychiatric Assessment		[ ]	[ ]	[ ]	
Psychological "		[ ]	[ ]	[ ]	incl. family/carer
GP NH Assessment		[ ]	[ ]	[ ]	
GP Medical "		[ ]	[ ]	[ ]	
GP Prescription only		[ ]	[ ]	[ ]	
Community Nurse: DN/ HV/PN		[ ]	[ ]	[ ]	
MH SW: Assessment		[ ]	[ ]	[ ]	
Therapy		[ ]	[ ]	[ ]	
Other SW: Assessment		[ ]	[ ]	[ ]	
Therapy		[ ]	[ ]	[ ]	
Home help		[ ]	[ ]	[ ]	
Day care		[ ]	[ ]	[ ]	
Support Groups: client		[ ]	[ ]	[ ]	
carer		[ ]	[ ]	[ ]	
Private agencies		[ ]	[ ]	[ ]	specify ....
Other services		[ ]	[ ]	[ ]	specify ....

Costs: Indirect

	£	
Cost of time off work for relatives	[ ]	(in 3 months)
Cost of time off work for patient	[ ]	
Cost of voluntary/private home help	[ ]	
Cost of mental health prescriptions	[ ]	
Cost of voluntary/private/day care/rehabilitation	[ ]	
Cost of fares for treatment	[ ]	
Extra cost of utilities (heating, lighting, food, resulting from patient care	[ ]	
Unforeseen costs specify:	[ ]	
Telephone calls	[ ]	
Costs of police contacts specify:	[ ]	

Costs: Community

	£	
Sickness/Invalidity benefit	[ ]	(in 3 months)
Supplementary benefit	[ ]	
Unemployment benefit	[ ]	
Attendance allowance	[ ]	
Mobility allowance	[ ]	
Single pension	[ ]	
Other public funding	[ ]	

Benefits

(1) Earnings

Earnings: Taking into account all the earnings coming into
the home after tax, which figure below comes closest to (i)
patient's, (ii) the family's income? Stress that this
information is strictly confidential and cannot be given to
any agency, e.g. Social Security, Tax Office, etc. Give this
page to carer to circle appropriate codes. Subsequent
assessments ask if any changes.

Weekly	or	Annual	Code	
			Patient	Family
No income		No income	0	0
Less than £21		Less than £1000	1	1
£21–40		£1001–2000	2	2
£41–60		£2001–3000	3	3
£61–80		£3001–4000	4	4
£81–100		£40001–5000	5	5
£101–120		£5001–6000	6	6
£121–140		£6001–7000	7	7
£111–160		£7001–8000	8	8
£161–180		£8001–9000	9	9
£181–200		£9001–10,000	10	10
£201–240		£10,001–12,000	11	11
£241–300		£12,001–15,000	12	12
£301–400		£15,001–20,000	13	13
Over £400		Over £20,000	14	14

(2) Hours of voluntary/sheltered work done per week   [   ]
specify ....

Administrative: Assessment completed   [   ]
                  Forms completed   [   ]
                  Reliability checked   [   ]
                  Management plan approved   [   ]
                  GP record completed   [   ]

Index

Italic page numbers refer to tables and figures

317

318

Strategies—*continued*
  for recurrence prevention,
    casework, 218–19
  to help drug compliance,
    193
  used in integrated mental
    health services, 20–3
Stress
  ambient, definition and
    approach, 31
  by carers of disabled people, 37
  and crisis intervention, 164–5
  factors, and recurrence of
    disorders, 188–90
  long-term disablement, 227
  management, 36–7
    and drug compliance, 198
    and early warning signs, 208
    in schizophrenic disorders,
      80–1
    training, 210
  onset, and onset of florid
    episode, time between,
    190
  pattern of physiological
    change, 31–6
  -related disorders
    strategies, 64, 65
    see also Adjustment disorders
  responses, mediation, 33
  –vulnerability model, 28–37
    see also Vulnerability-stress
Structuring sessions about the
    disorders, 204
Suicide
  assessment of risk factors, 111
  attempts, example, 212
  risk
    in depressive disorders, 76
    early detection, 111–14
    managing, home-based
      intensive care, 184–6
    procedures, 185–6
Supervised residential care,
    community-based
    mental health services,
    51

Surveys, epidemiological, to
    assess need, 5–8
Sydney Project, intensive care
    programs, 142–4

Tardive dyskinesia, management,
    79–80
Target problems
  dimensions for rating severity,
    169
  monitoring progress, 167–70
Team review
  initial, 260–1
  subsequent, 261–3
Teamwork model for community-
    based mental health
    care, 248–50
Temple University comparative
    study of behaviour
    therapy and psycho-
    therapy, 64
Test, Mary Ann, 47
Therapeutic strategies, effective,
    see Effective therapeutic
    strategies
Therapists
  cultural background
    differences, 125
  see also Mental health staff:
    Psychiatric consulta-
    tion: Staff
Time, mental health staff,
    allocation, 280–2
Training
  by all members of clinical
    team, 291
  communication, to prevent
    recurrence, 211–12
  in Community Living
    program, *141*
  in community living skills,
    235–8
    major areas, *236*
  family practice and mental
    health staff to conduct
    reliable assessments,
    104–10